On Your Bike
Essex

Tessa West

COUNTRYSIDE BOOKS
NEWBURY, BERKSHIRE

First published 2000
© Tessa West 2000
New Edition 2008

COUNTRYSIDE BOOKS
3 Catherine Road
Newbury, Berkshire

To view our complete range of books,
please visit us at
www.countrysidebooks.co.uk

ISBN 978 1 84674 127 2

Designed by Graham Whiteman
Photographs by the author
Maps by CJWT Solutions
Front cover picture Cyclographic Publications

Produced through MRM Associates Ltd., Reading
Printed in Thailand

CONTENTS

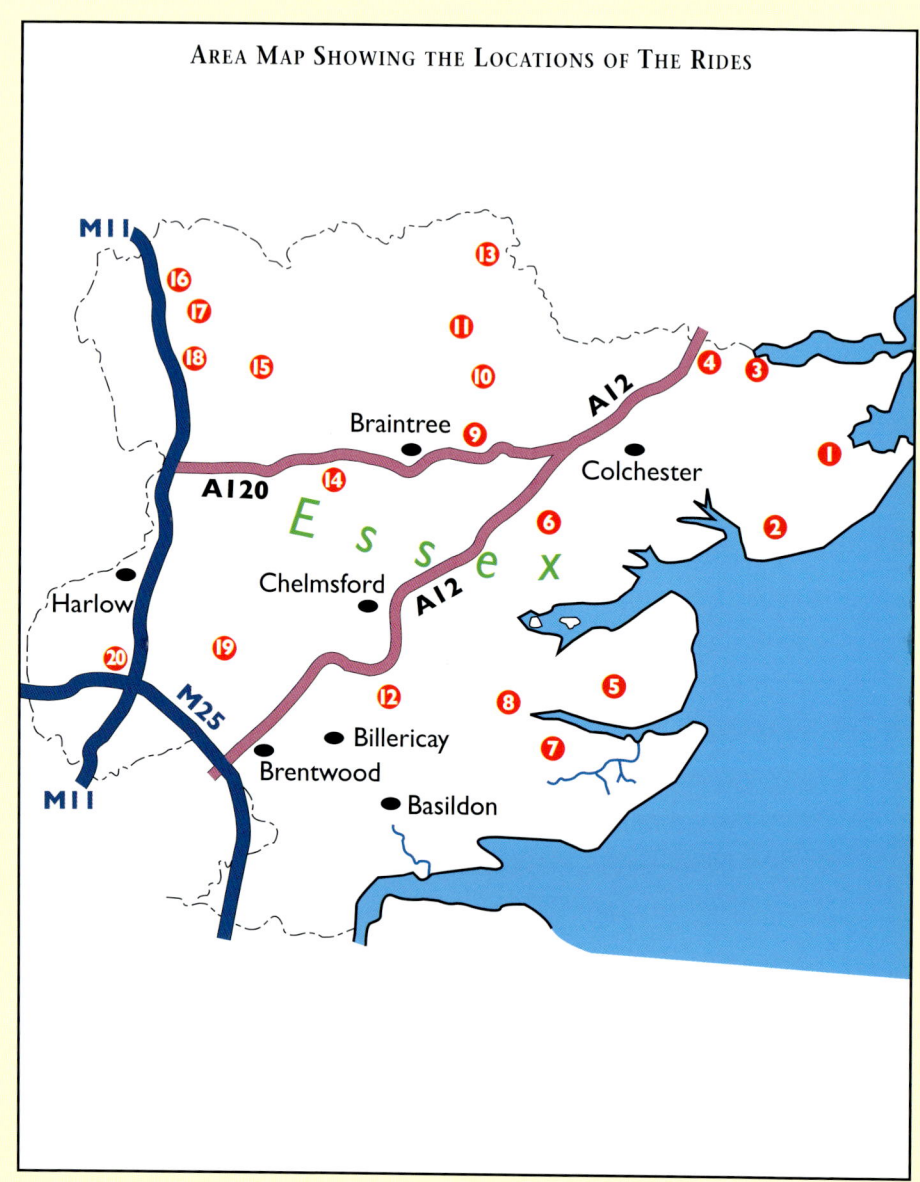

AREA MAP SHOWING THE LOCATIONS OF THE RIDES

INTRODUCTION

This book will help you to explore some of the beautiful places of Essex: wide sweeps of countryside, delicious villages, few real hills and plenty of rivers and coastline. The twenty rides will provide you with evidence of where people have been building, fighting, fishing and farming for two millennia, and some will take you into surprisingly remote places. You won't be bored.

Cycling is an excellent way to see the area. These rides take you round in a circular route so you end up where you started, and their intention is that you enjoy what you see and are pleased with the distance you have covered. Your attention is drawn to pubs, churches, jetties and a whole range of interesting features, but the road will hold other surprises you don't expect: a hawk swooping on its prey, an old fashioned barge in full sail, an ice cream van just where you want it.

Essex supports a large population, and few of these rides go into the heavily built up areas where most people live. But remarkably close to those large towns is beautiful countryside, and if you are a town dweller you could be out on your bike and away within an hour. Try a trip to Essex's muddy coastline, to a watermill, or to an ancient barn or monument. Keep an eye open for wildlife too. Take a picnic perhaps and treat yourself to a pub supper when you've finished.

The lengths of these routes vary from 11 to 22 miles. None of them is arduous to anyone who's reasonably fit. Older people and those who have not cycled recently are recommended to have a few rides closer to home before they tackle these. If you intend to take children with you, please see the relevant comments in the **Guide**. Almost everyone, even without trying, cycles at about ten miles an hour. It really is easy to cover the miles and, even if you want to stop every hour for ten minutes and then take a longer break to watch the world go by, a route of 20 miles should only take you around three and a half hours.

The whole point of this sort of cycling is enjoyment. So, if you don't like riding up a slope when you're tired – don't. Walk and push instead. If you are flagging, stop and rest or eat something. If the person you are with notices something they want to investigate, stop and have a look. Just take the book and set off and see what happens.

Good luck!

Tessa West

GUIDE TO USING THIS BOOK

Each route is preceded by information to help you:

The **route title** tells you the main places that you will start from or pass through. Please note that distances from nearby towns are as-the-crow-flies mileages. They are to help you find the starting place and are not true road distances. Because some cyclists will arrive at the starting point by car each route starts and ends in the same place. However, it is of course possible to start and finish the route wherever you want.

The **number of miles** is the total for the ride. Apart from a couple of rides which include short distances to be ridden on tracks, all the rides are on roads with hard surfaces.

The brief **introduction** to the ride gives a broad picture of where the route goes and also mentions particular features that you will see. The introduction is where you will find out whether the route takes you across or along any main roads.

The **maps** listed at the beginning of each ride are all Ordnance Survey maps in the Landranger series and it is advisable to take them with you as the sketch maps (see below) give limited information.

The **starting point** names a particular place in a village or town – including its grid reference – and gives its location in Essex in relation to other towns and, in some cases, to main roads.

Places for refreshment, sometimes particular pubs or tearooms, are mentioned in the pre-ride information, but you will find more places listed in the text about the ride. And others are just waiting for you to discover them. Don't forget Paragraph 211 of the Highway Code: You MUST NOT ride under the influence of drink or drugs.

Very few rides in this area are really hilly, but some indication is given about **ups and downs**.

THE ROUTES

It is a good idea to read right through a route before setting out so that you note any places where you want to spend more time. The routes have been arranged according to their position in Essex rather than their length or difficulty, so just choose ones you like the look of.

Each route itself is set out in blocks of only a few lines. This is so you can find your way around the page easily. The directions have been written as clearly as possible. Instructions to turn left or right are printed in bold, like this: **Turn L** at the T-junction; **bear R** when the road forks by the church. Instructions to continue straight over a crossroads or carry straight on are not in bold.

The directions include some description, but at the end of each route there is more information about **places of interest**. These include notes about architecture, history, legends and people.

The map of Essex on page 4 shows where the twenty routes are situated. Each individual route is accompanied by a simple **sketch map**. These maps are intended to give you a general idea of where the routes go but are not detailed enough to be route guides.

SAFETY
Safe bikes
Make sure that your bike and those of any companions – especially children – are roadworthy. This book is about routes not repairs, so seek elsewhere for do-it-yourself information or a good bike mechanic. It is silly to set off knowing that, say, your gears are not working properly or your saddle is too low. Get things checked before you go, especially if you are riding an unfamiliar bike.

Decide in advance what you are going to do if your bike gets a puncture, and be prepared. There is no point in equipping yourself with a puncture outfit if you don't know how to use it. It might be better to take a spare inner tube – plus the tools you'll need – but of course you'll need to know how to deal with this, too. A mobile phone might be the best insurance policy, assuming that there is someone to phone who is prepared to come and rescue you.

Make sure you don't have things dangling off handlebars or panniers.

Locking your bike will be completely unnecessary in most of the places these routes will take you to, but use your common sense and lock if in doubt.

Safe cycling
Wear comfortable clothes and shoes. Wear a helmet.

Stop if you want to consult a map or this book, otherwise you may ride into a car or a ditch.

If you are with someone else or a group make sure that the pace suits everyone or that you arrange that those who are ahead will stop at intervals to give the others time to catch up and get their breath before setting off again. If you are one of the fastest don't forget that the people behind you may not be so fit, so practised or so fond of cycling as you are. Look after them, and especially look after children who will certainly ride at a slower pace and will need more stops.

There are several places where the route includes a couple of miles of main road or where you need to cross a main road. You may feel safer if you walk and push your bike, particularly where there is a pavement, even if you extend your journey by half an hour.

Riding after dark is dangerous even with lights. Be very careful if you do it.

Children
Even if children are very used to cycling they are likely to get tired or fed up faster and they will be more at risk than most adults. They may make the wrong decision about a manoeuvre, their attention may be drawn to things off the road and they may decide to speed on ahead of you – or, more often, lag behind.

Hills will be harder work for them than adults. All in all, these rides will be quite a challenge to any child unless he or she is a fit teenager, so think twice before taking them.

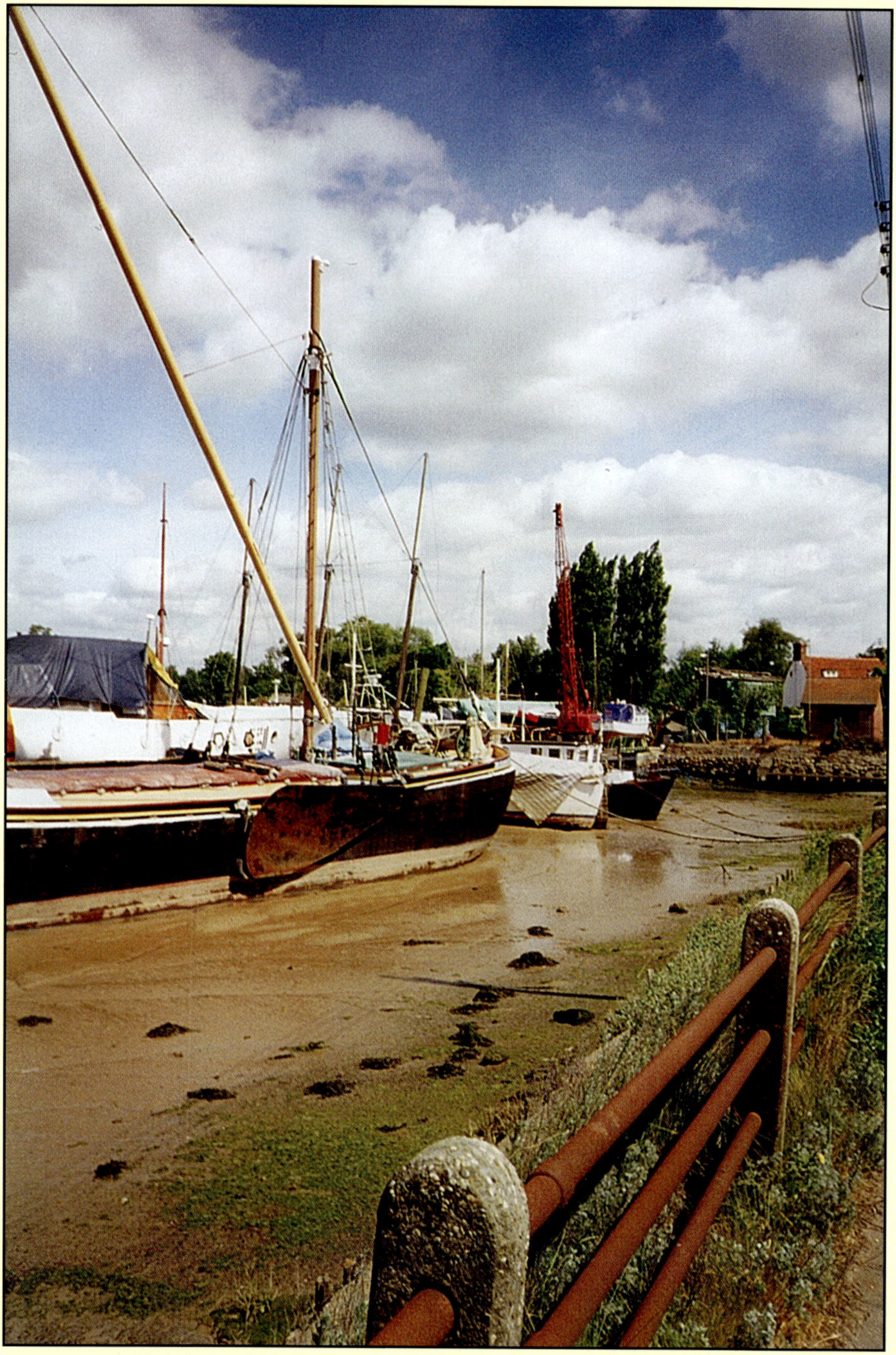

1

Thorpe-le-Soken, Great Oakley and Tendring

17 miles

This ride goes through soft landscapes where you see pastures and churches, substantial traditional houses and old farm buildings. It also gives you a glimpse of one of Essex's muddy estuaries which used to be busy with boats. It's hard to believe that these peaceful places are only a few miles from popular Walton-on-the-Naze and its neighbouring and more gentle resort, Frinton.

Notice, as you go along, the names of villages and farms: you'll go to Weeley and Wix, past Skighaugh and Dengewell Hall. Try to imagine what it must have been like to travel around here a hundred years ago on the most common form of transport – horseback.

Map: OS Landranger 169 Ipswich and The Naze.

Starting point: The Black Boy pub at Weeley (GR 147225). This is less than a mile from the A133, on the B1033. Weeley is about 7 miles north of Clacton-on-Sea and 12 miles east of Colchester. Parking is available at the Black Boy for patrons but please ask before leaving your car while you ride.

You'll be spoilt for choice for pubs on this route. There's the Black Boy for a start (and the finish), and you'll pass the Cherry Tree Inn, the Rose and Crown, the Bell, the Maybush, the Waggon at Wix and more. Great Oakley or Wix would be good midway places for something to eat.

This route has some hills but there's nothing too daunting. And most of it is flat. Even the B roads can be busy in summer, so take care.

Come out of the Black Boy car park and **turn L** onto the B1033. **Turn L** again at the duckpond, towards Tendring. After 2 miles **turn R** at the T-junction by the Cherry Tree Inn onto the B1035.

Stay on the B1035 until it joins the B1033 which takes you into Thorpe-le-Soken. Go along the High Street, past the church on your right, and **turn L** at the roundabout onto the B1414 towards Harwich.

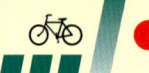

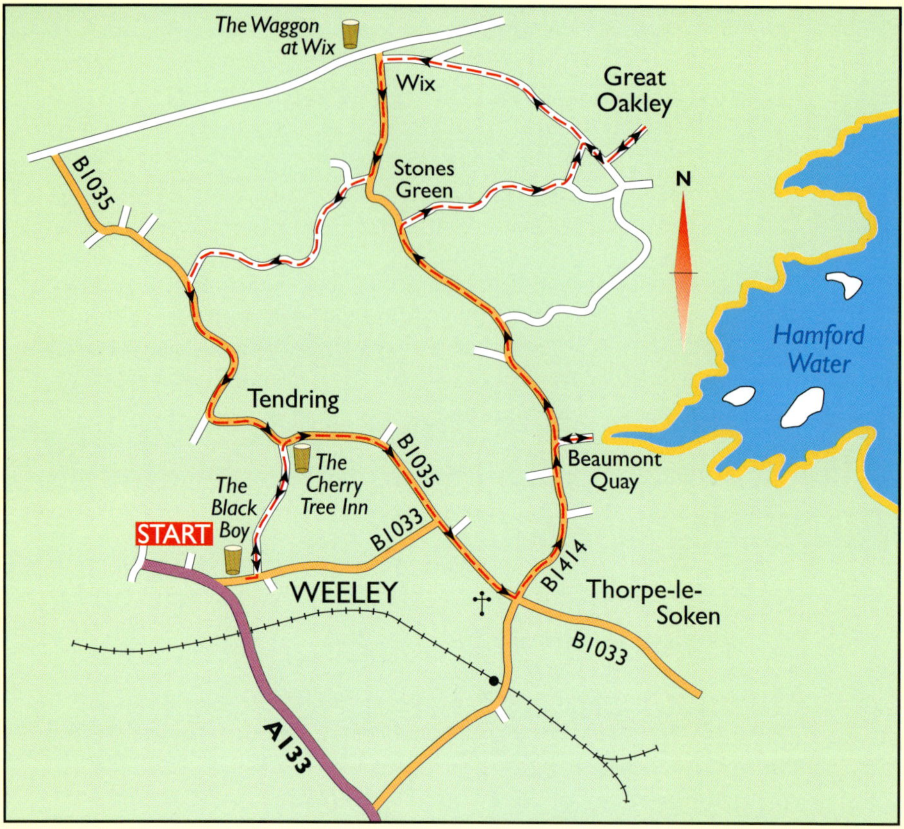

The Waggon at Wix

Wix

Great Oakley

B1035

Stones Green

N

Hamford Water

Tendring

B1035

The Cherry Tree Inn

The Black Boy

START

B1033

Beaumont Quay

B1414

WEELEY

Thorpe-le-Soken

B1033

A133

Go past Tendring Technical College before you are out of Thorpe and look ahead to a wonderful panorama. Look right and you'll see the sea – or at least the estuary of Hamford Water.

After a mile you pass, on your right, the turning to the B1034 to Walton. Ignore this but **turn R** at the next small road. This leads only to two farms. Ride up to the houses and park your bike in the Beaumont Quay car park on your right. Walk down to the quay and around the end to see the rotting hulk.

Go along the path for five minutes to see typical East Coast mud, birds and the sea beyond. In 20 minutes you can reach the beautiful little row of houses at Landermere Quay.

Back on your bike, ride up to the road you were on and **turn R**. Keep going for a mile or two and pass the sign for Beaumont-cum-Moze, keeping on the B1414. **Turn L** onto Wix Road, towards Stones Green.

As you enter this tiny hamlet you begin to see signs telling you this is Route 51 of the National Cycle

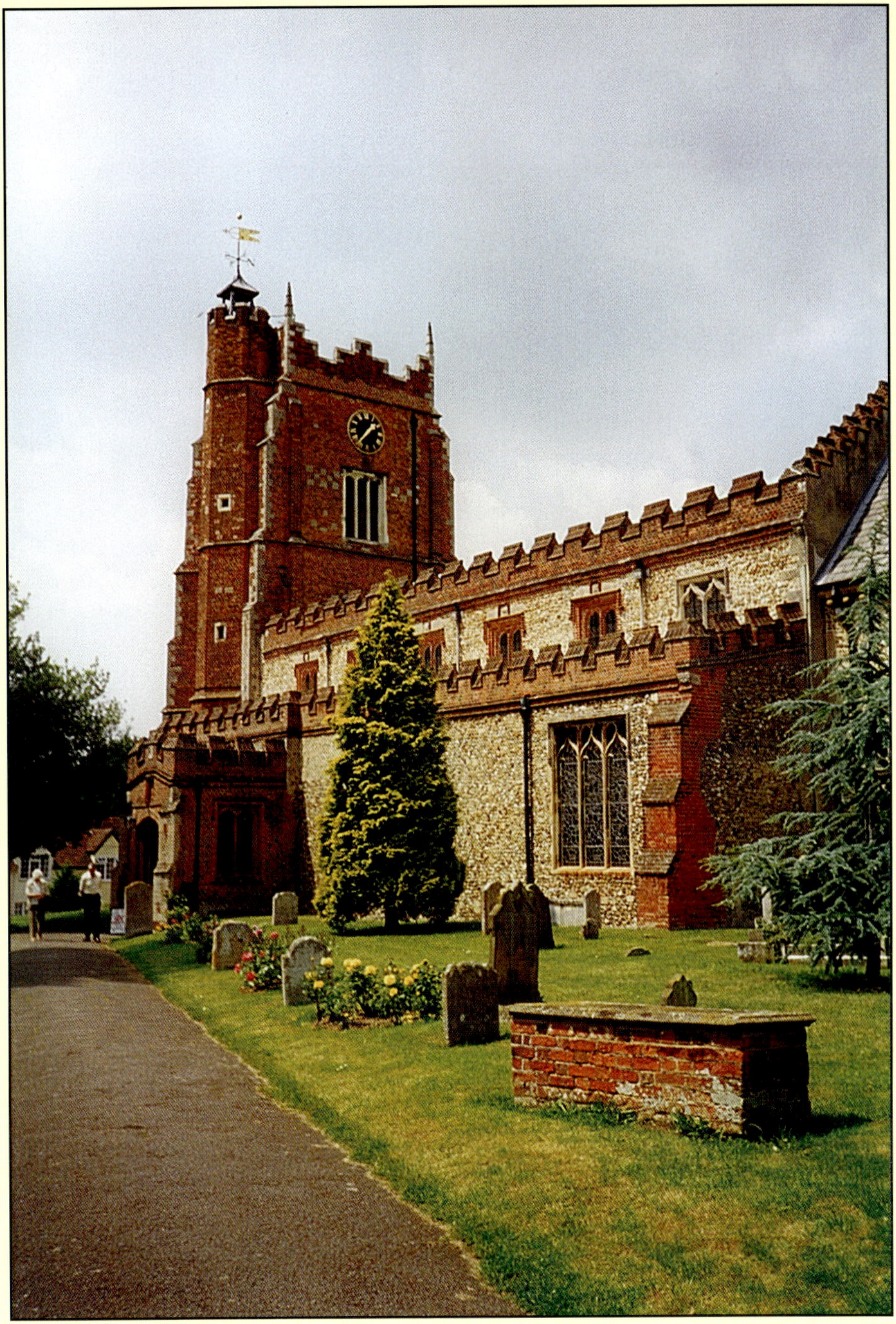

Thorpe-le-Soken church

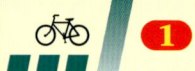
Network. After 1½ miles **turn sharp R** into Stones Green Road and continue for a good 2 miles **bearing L** at the only junction (with Red Barn Lane) until you see Great Oakley church on your right.

Turn R at the T-junction, and then **L** into Great Oakley. It's worth riding past the shop and along to the little square with the war memorial and the Maybush pub.

Then retrace your wheel marks back to the junction where you **turn R**, along the road you came from, signposted to Wix. But instead of taking the road back to Stones Green, carry straight on, following the National Cycle Network signs, and continue to Wix.

After about 1½ miles you reach Harwich Road. **Turn L** and the White Hart is on your right. Continue along here until you come to the next crossroads. **Turn L** at the ancient looking Waggon at Wix pub. Ride on for a mile until you see the sign for Great Bentley.

Turn R at the little triangular junction towards Little Bentley. Then, within a couple of hundred yards, **turn L** down a little lane.

You will come to the B1035 where you **turn L** by the Tendring post office towards Clacton.

Continue along here, past the school with its distinctive roof on your right, and follow the road at a sharp bend to the left by Tendring church.

Ride for ½ mile or so until you reach the Cherry Tree Inn. **Turn R** here, and ride back into Weeley. **Turn R** when you reach the B1033 and the Black Boy is on your right.

● ●

THORPE-LE-SOKEN

The church here is well worth a visit. Its red brick tower, red tiled roof and rambling, verdant chuchyard make it the perfect place for a rest. But there has been drama here. In the 1700s the vicar's young bride, Kitty Canham, decided that village life was too boring, so she ran away to London. She met and bigamously married a wealthy lord who took her around Europe for four years. But she became ill and when she realised she was dying she confessed in writing that she was already married and that she wanted to be buried back in Thorpe-le-Soken. The lord brought her body back and one story records that he stood side by side at the graveside with her first husband, who forgave them both, while another suggests that he was arrested when he arrived in England with the coffin. Kitty's ghost is said, perhaps not surprisingly, to haunt the Bell pub.

BEAUMONT QUAY

This derelict little quay, built with stones from the old London Bridge, was once full of boats that made their way up the creeks from Hamford Water at high tide with goods from

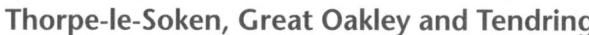 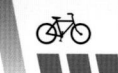

London and the Continent. Its remoteness made it a smugglers' delight. Amongst the mudflats near here is an island which has an explosives factory and is joined to the mainland by a causeway. Arthur Ransome's book *Secret Water* is based on Hamford Water. On a clear day The Naze is visible on the horizon.

TENDRING
The Tendring hundred (a hundred is a sub-division of a county or region) consisted of over thirty villages, of which Tendring village was the centre. The church here is dedicated to St Edmund, the king of East Anglia who was killed by the Danes and buried at Bury St Edmunds. Built of stone and rubble, the church has an ancient and elegant wooden porch.

Great Bentley, St Osyth and Point Clear

16 miles

This is a real mixture of a route. It starts in Great Bentley, the most tranquil of villages, leads you to St Osyth, past an ancient abbey, and on to Point Clear with its seaside caravan sites and sticks of rock. The ride back to the north takes you through gentle, quiet countryside.

So this ride gives you a chance to sit on a beach, see a martello tower that's been turned into a museum, admire little weatherboarded houses and get a feel for the sea and boats. You'll come across the story of a sloop, scarcely longer than the width of an ordinary road, in which a sailor from St Osyth circumnavigated the world in the late 1980s.

Map: OS Landranger 169 Ipswich and The Naze.

Starting point: Great Bentley railway station (GR 112214) on the road to St Osyth and Clacton where there is a free car park. Great Bentley is 7 miles east of Colchester, and 9 miles north-west of Clacton-on-Sea.

Great Bentley has a pub – the Plough – and there are more in St Osyth. Point Clear has the modern Ferryboat Inn, and several other various places for refreshment, some of which could be said to have traditional seaside character. On the way home you'll pass the Beehive.

Bits of this route are busy, especially in holiday times. You need to go on the B1027 and on two occasions you will have to cross at busy places. It's therefore not a good ride for children.

Come out of the railway station and **turn L** across the level crossing. Stay on this minor road to St Osyth and you reach Aingers Green, but do not turn L here. Just keep going, ignoring a turn to the right.

When you reach a T-junction **turn L** onto the B1027. Be careful, for this is a busy road. The Flag pub is on the right. Just go straight on and in 2 miles you will reach St Osyth.

It may be safest to stop, get off your bike and push it across the road when you **turn R** onto a minor road and into St Osyth. Ride for ½ mile into the centre (there's a deer park on your right) and carefully **turn R** at a tricky crossroads, following signs to Point Clear and the abbey.

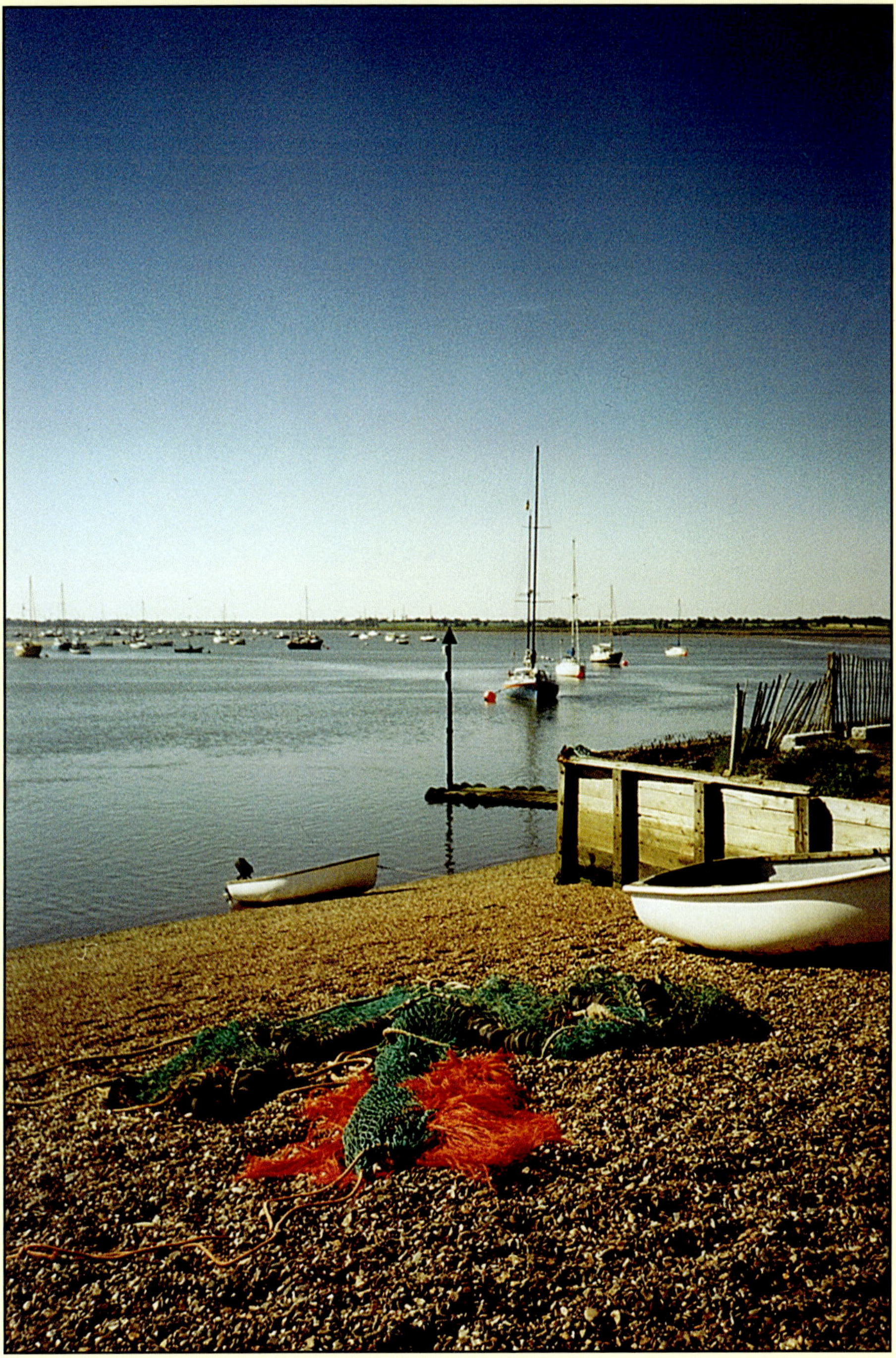

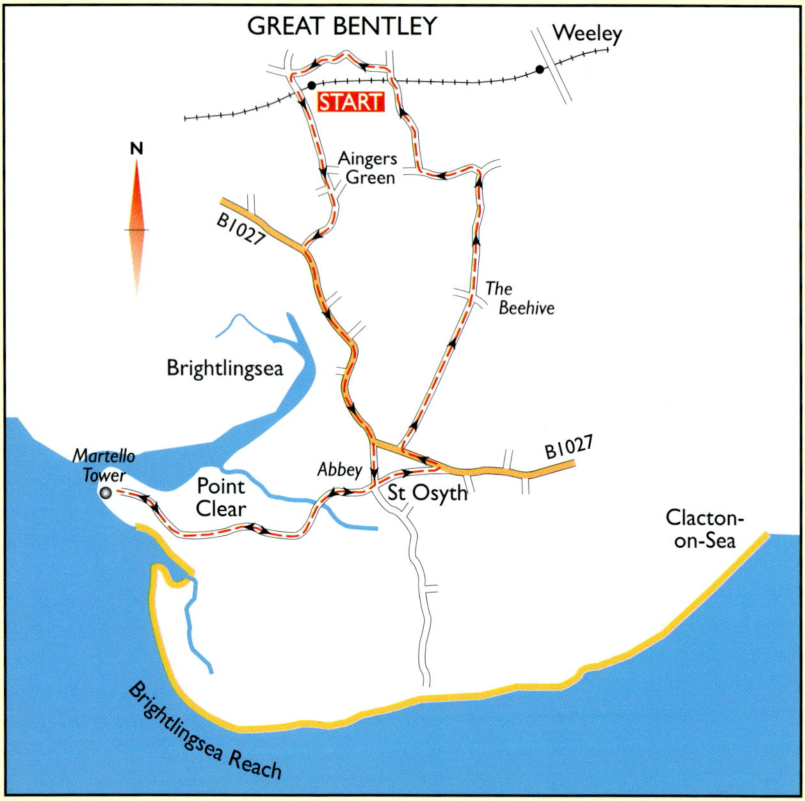

GREAT BENTLEY

Weeley

START

Aingers
Green

B1027

N

The
Beehive

Brightlingsea

Martello
Tower

Abbey

Point
Clear

St Osyth

B1027

Clacton-
on-Sea

Brightlingsea Reach

Ride along here, leaving the impressive abbey on your right, and continue past the playing field and the White Hart and then down across the causeway over the St Osyth Creek where there are masts and sizeable boats on one side and swans and little boats on the other.

Follow the road round a sharp R-hand bend and on for a couple of miles until the surburban type houses give way to less substantial holiday homes and then to caravans. When you reach the roundabout with a big notice,

Orchard Holiday Park, you know you're in Point Clear.

Bear L along the Eastern Promenade and follow signs to the Ferryboat Inn. There's a rising green on your left, with the beach beyond. Continue through the caravan site until you come to the heart of Point Clear: You'll find the martello tower which houses the East Essex Aviation Museum, the Ferryboat Inn, a small amusement arcade and a shop or two.

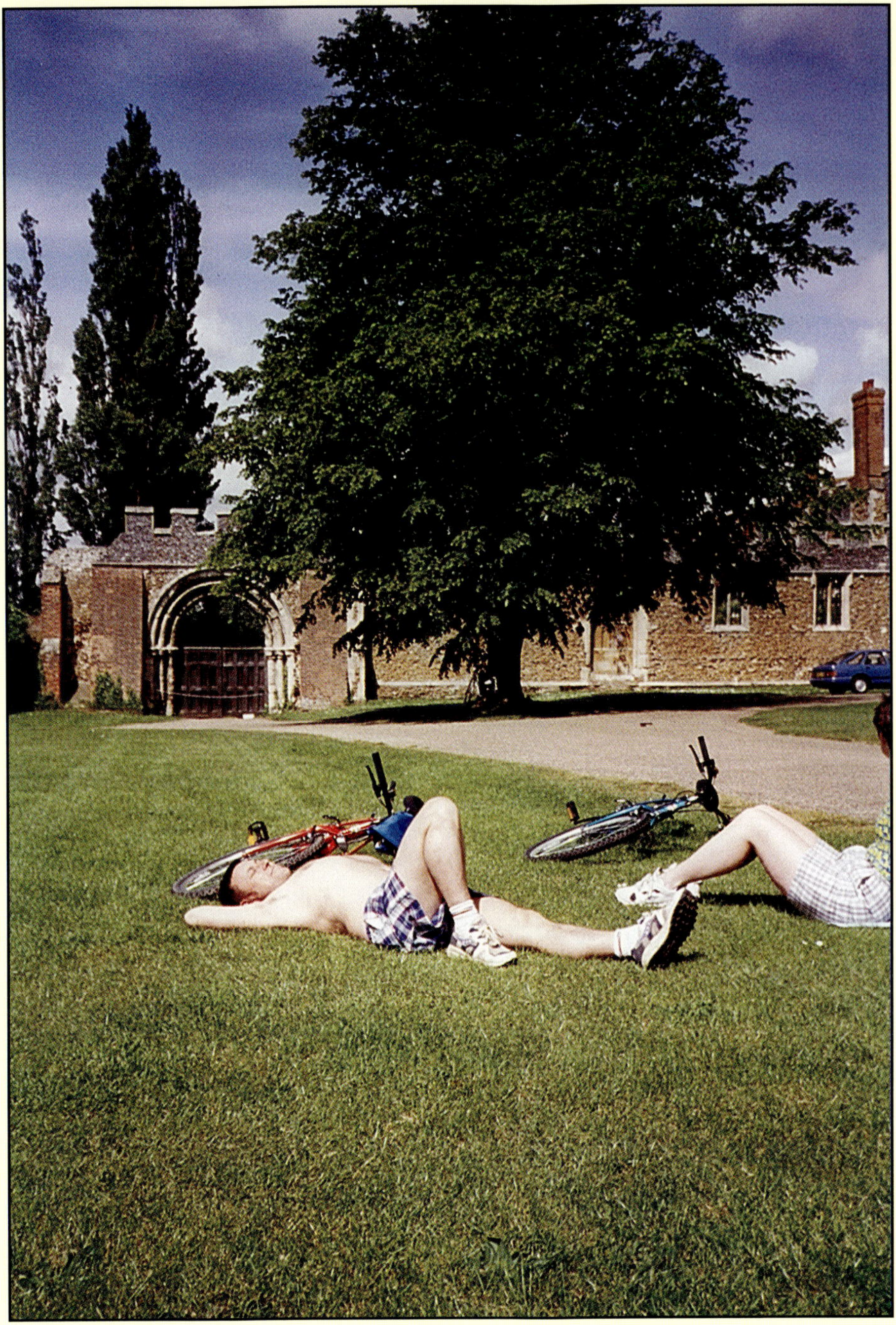

Taking a break outside the abbey at St Osyth

If you go even further along you come to a stretch of sand and mud that gives you a view of a flotilla of small boats bobbing on the tide (if it's in) and across to Brightlingsea.

Then you must turn around and head back along the same road out of Point Clear and back to St Osyth. Note, as you pass the abbey, the plaque on the other side of the road commemorating Trevor Osben's single-handed sail round the world.

Go straight across the crossroads towards Clacton-on-Sea, but note St Osyth's interesting little houses. It also has several shops which look as if they sell everything. Ride on for a few hundred yards then **turn L** into St Claire's Street. Ride to the end and go between the concrete bollards onto the main road.

This is the busy B1027 again, so take care. **Turn L** onto it and then almost immediately **R** into Clay Road towards Weeley. It might be best to dismount and walk across here by the cemetery on the corner.

Continue along this straight and quiet road for 1½ miles and then go straight over the minor crossroads by the Beehive. Ride on for just over 1 mile, partly under leafy arches, until you reach a T-junction.

Turn L here, and then after a further ½ mile, **turn R** onto a road indicating Great Bentley and Tendring.

Ride along this quiet road for 1½ miles. Ignore the first turn to the left but when you have crossed over the railway bridge, **turn L** onto Weeley Road towards Great Bentley. You will be back where you started in about 2 miles.

• •

GREAT BENTLEY

The most noticeable fact about Great Bentley is its huge 43 acre village green – the biggest in England. History shows that, despite an early incident in which five local people were burned at the stake in Colchester for their religious beliefs, the village later supported a variety of denominations who respected each other and maintained a spirit of independence in defending their green from a range of development proposals.

During the Second World War the closed level crossing was the site of a serious dispute between the stationmaster and an officer trying to get across with an American Airforce ambulance. The officer threatened to shoot the lock or the stationmaster but did neither as the expected express train roared through in the nick of time.

ST OSYTH

Osyth was the daughter of the first Christian king of the East Angles and she founded a nunnery here. When she refused to worship the pagan gods of a group of marauding Danes they beheaded her and a spring of water rose from the ground.

The most outstanding feature of St Osyth is the 14th century abbey, or priory, of St Clere's Hall. Its imposing gatehouse is set back from the road, fronted by a huge tree and a green, with a large deer park behind. It's a sound, solid building that was assaulted in the Civil War by a mob of Puritans. Unfortunately neither the priory nor park are open to the public at present.

POINT CLEAR

This is a traditional place for Essex holidaymakers, so don't arrive expecting a quiet corner with the call of seabirds and a country pub. Take it as it is – a place for families to have a break from routine, to eat ice creams on beaches and to watch the lines of moored boats in Brightlingsea Creek. It'll provide a real contrast to the other places on this ride.

3

Manningtree, Mistley, Wrabness and Wix

14 miles

This route runs parallel with the gentle estuary of the River Stour which is within view for almost all of the outward journey. You can see across to the Shotley Peninsula and to the imposing Royal Hospital School. Mistley is an unexpectedly nautical little town where you'll see swans and sailing boats galore, and evidence of a once busy and still active port. It looks a peaceful scene, but in the 1600s a zealous witch hunter was rounding up women he found suspicious, holding trials and executing them. Don't let this put you off.

Map: OS Landranger 169 Ipswich and The Naze or 168 Colchester, Halstead and Maldon.

Starting point: Behind the Crown pub, The Quay, Manningtree (GR 106319). Manningtree is about 11 miles south-west of Ipswich and 9 miles north-east of Colchester. It's busy here in summer so if you fail to find a parking space by the river, try inland away from the river front.

There are several pubs in Mistley and Manningtree, and the Mistley Quay Café does coffees, teas and lunches. You'll ride past the Strangers Home pub in Bradfield and there are places for refreshment in Wrabness.

You need to ride on the B1352. In summer there can be a considerable amount of traffic and therefore this route is not suitable for children. Don't reverse this route because, amazingly, it has more downs than ups this way round.

Stand facing the river and the railway line beyond (visible only when there's a train) and **turn R** onto the road so that the river is on your left. Follow it along towards Mistley Towers, watching out for swans.

You are riding along The Walls and on your right is Mistley Place Park and its church. Then you reach Mistley Towers on your left.

On your left are the quayside and storage buildings and you could dip down to the left for a closer look. Keep going straight on and note the Mistley Quay Café and Swan

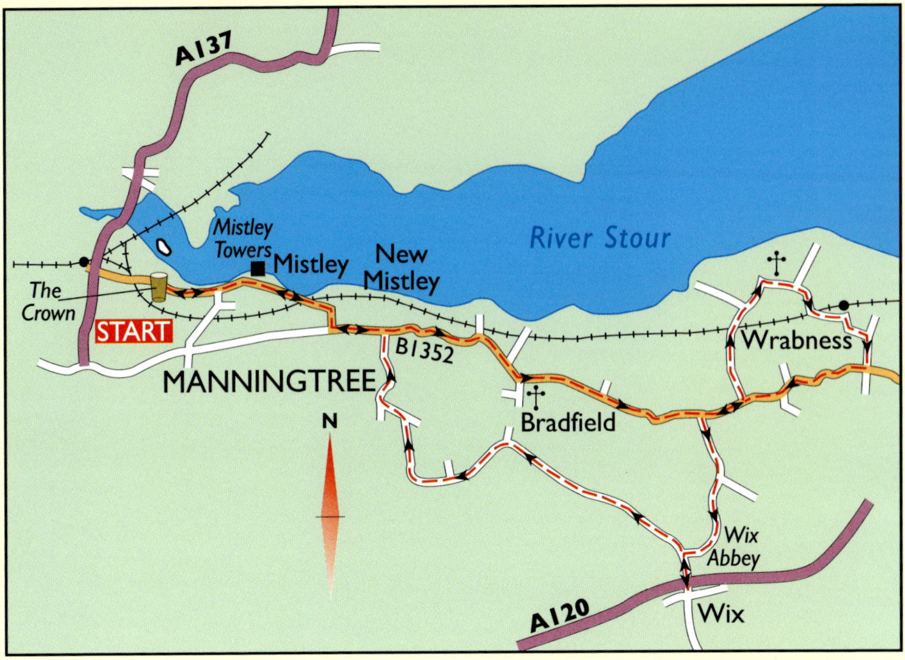

Fountain on your left. Then continue along, on to Harwich Road and over the railway.

The road bends by the Anchor Inn. Enjoy a stunning view of the Stour estuary as you descend into Bradfield.

Turn L at the Strangers Home pub at the corner by the square church towards Ramsey and Harwich and relax on a good run down before a manageable ride up. Be careful here because this bit of road can get busy. Note Jacques Hall and also the view over the Stour, both on your left.

Turn L into Wheatsheaf Lane and ride along a road which takes you under a railway bridge. You'll pass a green burial ground on your left in Oakfield Wood. Just stay on the road and on your left you will see, set on a wonderful site above the estuary, the church with its bells in a wooden cage.

Turn L at the T-junction by the railway bridge as you reach Wrabness and follow the road past the railway station, through the village and then down to the crossroads.

Turn R at the crossroads, back onto to the B1352. You come to Wheatsheaf Lane again. Ride past it and **turn L** ½ mile later, by Spinnel's Farm.

Ride along this quiet road and after 2 miles you reach a road junction by Abbey Farm. **Turn L** here and **L**

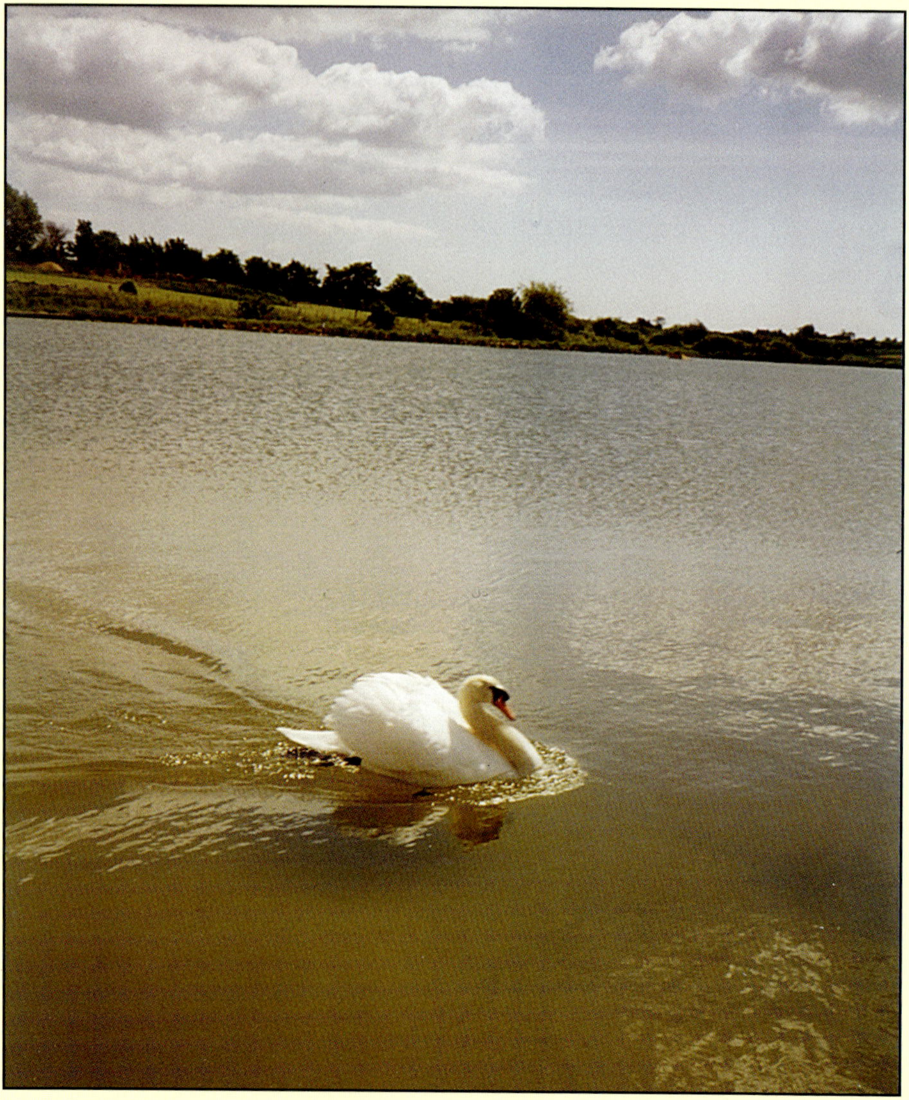

The River Stour

again into the driveway to get a taste of the church and former Wix Abbey.

When you are ready turn round and return to Abbey Farm. **Bear L** here, keeping on the road towards Bradfield. After 2½ miles **turn L** at the junction by the Village Maid pub.

Go through Bradfield Heath, heading in the direction of a tall

mast and passing the Methodist church on your right. Then **turn R** onto Straight Road which is signposted to Mistley Heath. Follow the road through Mistley Heath and back towards Mistley.

Turn L (onto the B1352 again) and then continue back past the Anchor Inn, Mistley railway station and the Mistley Quay Café before re-entering Manningtree.

● ●

MISTLEY

Mistley has been a busy port for generations. Once it imported coal, timber and horse manure and exported grain, bricks, flour and hay for horses. Ships went off to the Armada from docksides here. In the 1700s Richard Rigby developed it as a port with a difference: a new shipyard, quays, timber and coal yards, a limekiln and maltings. Simultaneously and equally ambitiously he converted an ordinary hall into a stately home – Mistley Hall – but he ran out of funds.

Another person well known in Mistley was Matthew Hopkins, the 17th century Witchfinder General. He found 194 witches, some of them local, and he

caused the horrific deaths of most of them. Today, swans give Mistley a much more serene image.

THE STOUR ESTUARY

The Stour is the border between Essex and Suffolk. John Constable painted river scenes within walking distance of Manningtree, and the estuary here is wide, tidal and full of interest. People were sailing up and down here 4,000 years ago and their successors are still doing so. As well as swans there are curlews, pintails, shelducks and dunlin. Even if you can't recognise these wildfowl you will notice their calls which are entirely different from land birds. Once samphire grew on the banks of the estuary and was valued because it could be either eaten or burnt to produce a soda used for glassmaking.

WIX ABBEY

Sometime around 1130 Henry I established 'an institution of a religious order for nuns for ever' in the already existing Priory of Wix. Henry VI confirmed this in 1438. The priory was visited by Bishop Fitz James in 1509, and he forbad the nuns there to permit any spectacles of 'javelin-play, dances or trading' or 'to wear silver or gilt hairpins'. So, make sure you behave in a seemly manner.

Dedham, Higham, Boxted and Langham

16 miles

This is a delightful rivery ride. You start off by Dedham Mill on the Stour and cross it northwards and southwards, moving from Essex to Suffolk and back again. You'll cross other streams too, each with their own little bridge. Don't forget to take bread for the ducks.

And on this ride you pass some outstandingly beautiful country houses and gardens of different periods and styles. In summer this is English countryside at its gentlest, greenest best and it understandably held appeal for one of the most famous English landscape painters, John Constable.

Note that Dedham itself can be packed in summer, but you will hardly be riding there.

Maps: OS Landranger 168 Colchester, Halstead and Maldon and 155 Bury St Edmunds, Sudbury and Stowmarket.

Starting point: The car park opposite Dedham Mill (GR 058335). Dedham Mill is on the B1029, just north of Dedham, on the Stour. Dedham is just off the A12 about 7 miles north of Colchester.

There's plenty of choice as regards refreshment. Dedham itself has pubs and tearooms, but a particularly good place to end is the Dedham Art and Craft Centre. Housed in a converted church this serves snacks and meals and has a fascinating toy museum. You will find other pubs en route but a riverside picnic might be a better idea.

Because rivers run downhill you'll be able to freewheel sometimes. Of course this means that you'll need to climb upwards too, but the views will reward you.

Start from the car park and **turn L** onto the B1029 into Dedham. Then **turn R** at the T-junction by the church, staying on the B1029 which is the main street.

A little way up the hill **turn R** into Stratford Road. Pass the Maison Talbooth Hotel on your left and then Milsoms on your right. Carry on and over the A12 and then **bear L** and soon **turn R** into Dedham

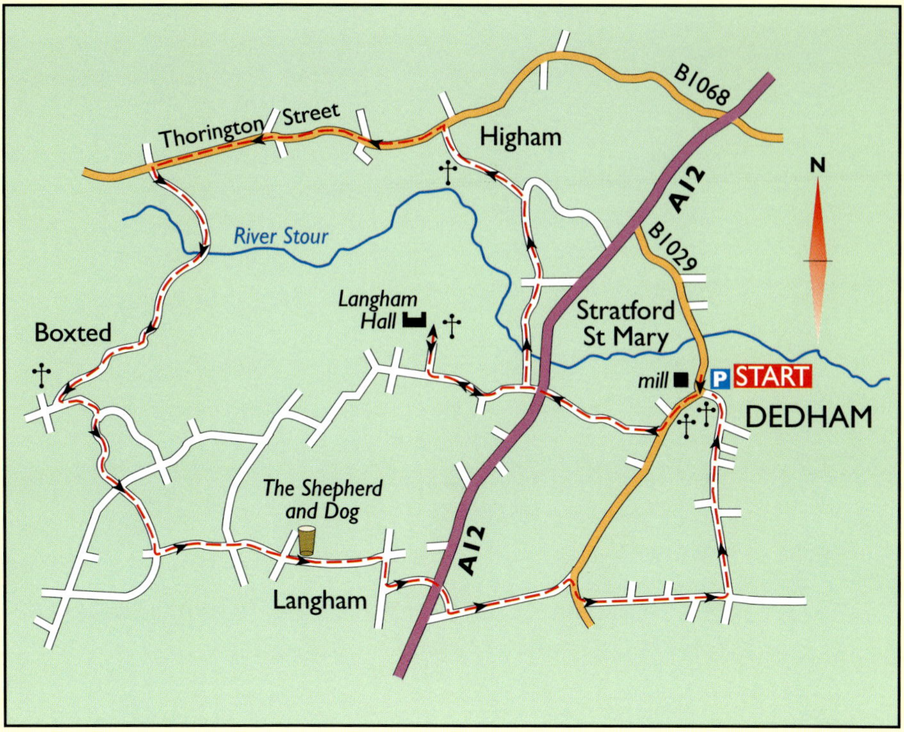

Road towards Langham. Then **turn R** down the driveway to Langham Hall and Langham church.

When you have admired the church in its pretty setting go back up the drive and **turn L** back the way you came and then **turn L** onto the road towards Stratford, signposted for Ipswich.

Keep straight on past the Tolbooth and the Black Horse (on the right). Stratford Lock and the waterworks are on the left. You are now in Stratford St Mary. Stay on this road (rather than going into the main part of Stratford) and at the small crossroads **turn L** towards Higham.

Continue – perhaps with a small detour down the drive to Higham church – until you reach the B1068 at Higham, by a triangular green. **Turn L** here towards Stoke-by-Nayland. After a mile or two you go through Thorington Street. Then **turn L** towards Boxted.

Ride down to a beautiful little bridge. Once over it you'll be back in Essex again. **Turn R**.

Continue into Boxted and follow the road round and through the village. The unusual church is set back on the right-hand side and is well worth a visit.

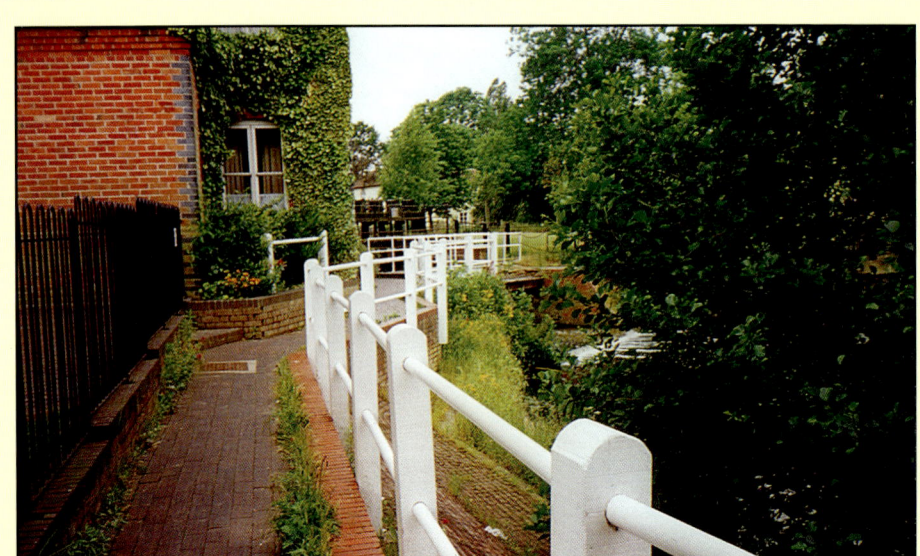

A walkway at Dedham Mill

Come out of the church and continue along to the T-junction. **Turn L** here towards Boxted Cross.

Ride down a steepish hill and then **turn R** at the bottom and up Carter's Hill.

Cross over the diagonal crossroads into Cage Road. After a few hundred yards **turn L** onto a small public bridleway. This is a beautiful little lane under trees and between deep banks. It is highly suitable for cyclists.

Turn L at the T-junction and then almost immediately **R** by the triangle of grass.

Keep straight on into Langham. Go straight over the crossroads by the Shepherd and Dog and then **turn R** at the T-junction.

Turn L into Birchwood Road. Cross the A12 again and **turn L** at the T-junction towards Dedham. You're still on Birchwood Road.

After a mile **turn R** at the crossroads towards Ardleigh on the B1029 and then, after a couple of hundred yards, **turn L** towards Lawford.

After another mile or so **turn L** at the crossroads and then ride back to Dedham past the Rose and Gown. As you come into Dedham there is a small lane on the left leading to Southfields and the Drift. **Turn L** here and enjoy an unusual and

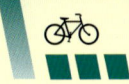
peaceful ride for the final few hundred yards back into Dedham, arriving by the church.

To reach Dedham Mill car park, cross over the main street and ride down the road (by the Marlborough Head) you came from at the start. The car park is down there on the right.

● ●

DEDHAM

This little town is well known because the artist John Constable went to its grammar school and painted the mill here. His painting of Flatford Mill, a couple of miles down the Stour towards the estuary, is even more famous. Dedham Mill has been converted into luxury flats but it's still there, and water still pours over the weir. The church is evidence of the wealth which was created by the weaving trade. Sherman's Hall, originally owned by the ancestors of General Sherman of the American Civil War, is another example of the profit from successful trade.

Dedham was also the home of another artist, Sir Alfred Munnings, whose house and studio are open to visitors.

BOXTED

Normans were the first to build the church of St Peter, but there have been many additions and alterations to it since then, including a surprisingly modern looking dormer window installed by the Tudors.

In 1906 the Salvation Army set up a Labour Colony here but there were problems with its administration and it was closed within ten years. Wartime in Boxted included a doodlebug and, on 30th August 1940, bombs. Some of the incendiaries failed to ignite and no one was hurt, but it was harvest time and as the priority was to protect the newly cut and stacked crops several labourers walked round the fields and put out the flames.

LANGHAM

This was a favourite place of Constable's because his friend the curate enabled him to have secret meetings at the rectory with the woman he loved. There's no memorial to these trysts but in the churchyard is a separate schoolroom with an interesting notice and in the porch is an old plaque that was once posted by the steep Gun Hill, exhorting drivers not to be cruel to their animals.

5

The Dengie Peninsula

21 miles

The Dengie Peninsula is basically made of land that becomes marshier and muddier the further east you go. Its northern and southern boundaries are the estuaries of the River Blackwater and the River Crouch. St Peter's chapel, a feature of this ride, looks out to the North Sea over the east coastline. This is a route where you'll see sails above fields and water where you don't expect it. It may seem far from modern England, but Bradwell Power Station is a reminder that it's not all seagulls and shelly beaches.

Map: OS Landranger 168 Colchester, Halstead and Maldon.

Starting point: The railway station at Southminster (GR 962996) where there is a free car park. Southminster is about 18 miles east of Chelmsford.

The Station Arms in Southminster is only a few minutes from your start and finish point. You'll pass the Cap and Feathers and the Fox and Hounds in Tillingham, plus a couple more pubs en route to Bradwell Waterside. On some weekends in summer, Eastlands Farm near St Peter's chapel does teas, but a picnic by the sea wall would be an excellent idea. You might even see a seal or two.

There's little that could be called hilly on this route, but be prepared for winds coming in off the sea. There is one section where you ride along the sea wall for about 3 miles, and although this is the most mild off-road riding you could find anywhere, it still takes more energy than riding along tarmac.

Ride out of the station car park and **turn L** onto the road leading into Southminster. **Turn R** onto the B1021, signposted to Tillingham. **Bear R** with the road you are on and continue out of Southminster.

Bear R at another sharp corner and continue into and through Asheldham. Keep straight on at the next road junction, following signs for Dengie and The Marshes. You'll pass a little church on your left and a Public Weighbridge on your right.

Keep straight on at the next

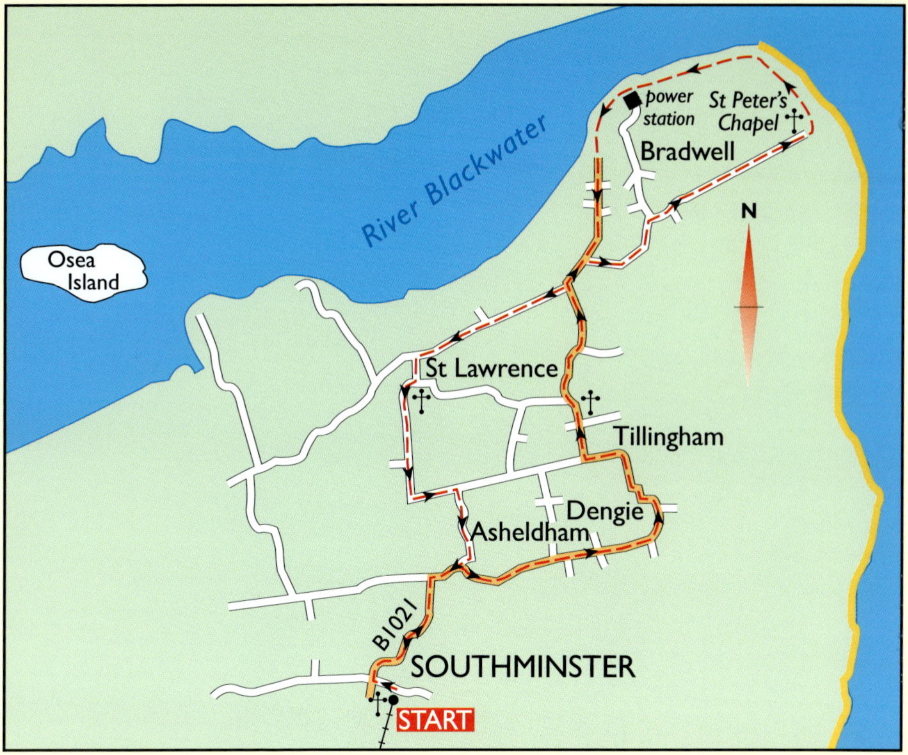

junction, ignoring the turn to the left. Follow this small road for a couple more miles, always **bearing left**, until you round a sharp **left hand bend** and the **turn R** towards Bradwell. Go along this street and you are in Tillingham. Pass the Cap and Feathers before reaching the village green with the Fox and Hounds, pretty weatherboarded houses and the church.

Stay on this road (still the B1021) and ride for a few miles. **Turn R** at the T-junction by a no longer used pub and continue into Bradwell-on-Sea. **Turn R** at the first turning to the right, signposted to St Peter's

chapel, and then **turn R** again by the church.

Ride on for 3 miles, through a housing estate and past the Cricketers and on along a former Roman road, past Eastlands Farm and along a wide track to St Peter's chapel.

When you have looked inside the chapel, push or ride your bike down past the chapel towards the sea until you reach the path along the sea wall. **Turn L** onto this. You can ride along here but you need to stop when you pass pedestrians.

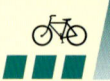

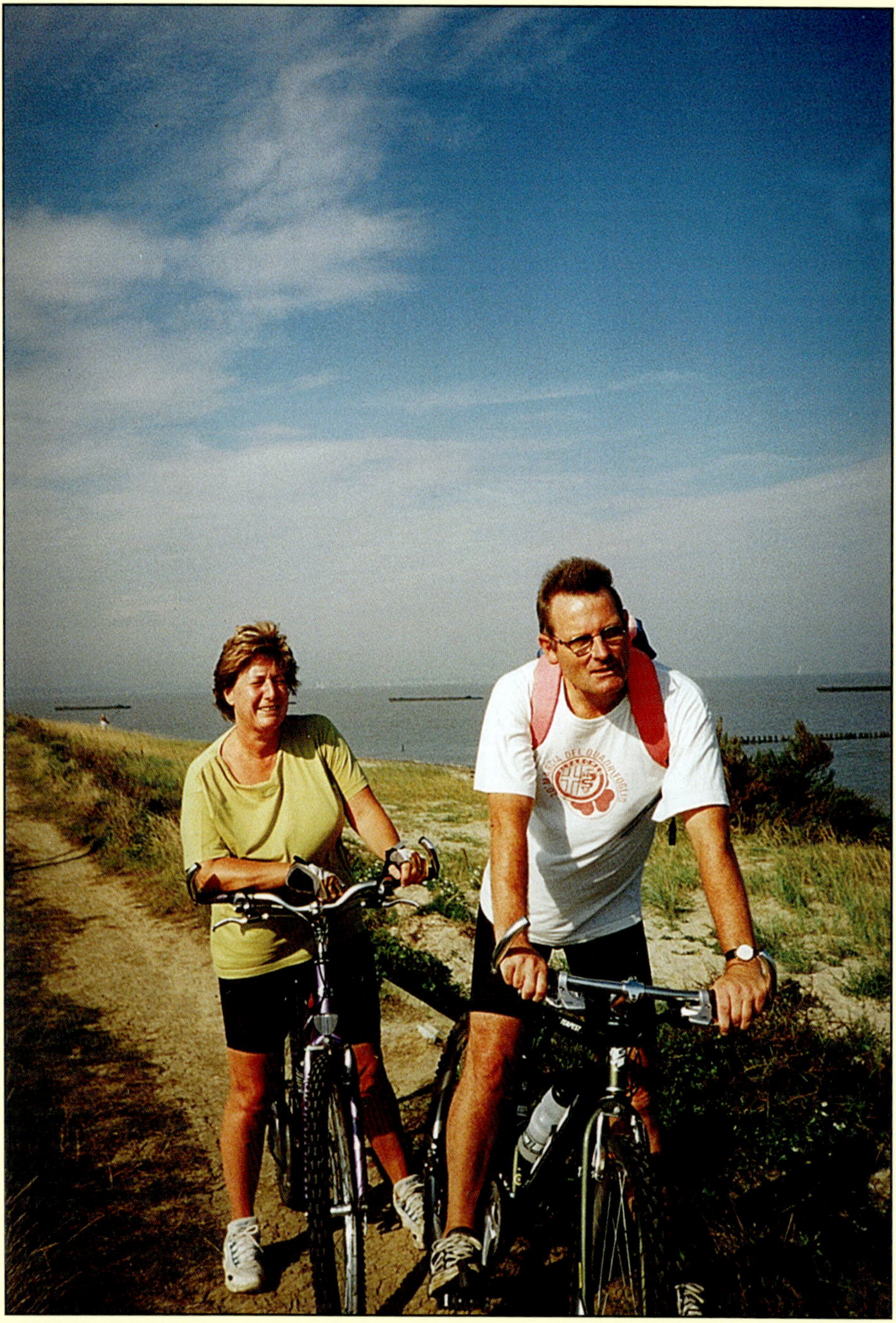

Cyclists on the sea wall

Follow this wall for about 3 miles, but do stop to admire the view and to walk down on to the beach which is virtually made of shells.

Keep going until you pass the huge, blocky power station. Once past it you are almost in Bradwell Marina.

Turn L off the path you have been riding on and up the road past the Green Man. Follow the road (this is the B1021 again) up and out of Bradwell. After 2 or 3 miles keep straight on – do not take the left turn to Tillingham.

Carry on along your small road for another few miles until you come to St Lawrence. **Turn L** up a small lane towards a church with a steeple. Then **turn R** and then **L**, signposted towards Asheldham.

After a couple of miles you ride round a sharp left-hand bend. After a further mile **turn R**, still heading for Asheldham. Once in Asheldham, continue along this road which takes you back into Southminster. It is the same road that you set out along.

•••••••••••••••••••••••••••••

SOUTHMINSTER
In the centre of Southminster stands St Leonard's church. It was started in Saxon times but has had substantial alterations carried out, particularly by the Victorians. A former vicar, Dr Scott, was chaplain to Admiral Lord Nelson on board *The Victory*, and there are several pieces of Nelson's . furniture from the ship in the church

today: a chart table, bookcase, chest commode and even a fireplace. Apparently Nelson died in Dr Scott's arms.

Above the porch is a room in which it is thought that monks from St Osyth's Priory, near Clacton, came to teach local children. The priory, or abbey, owned Southminster church from about 1120 to the Dissolution in 1540.

ST PETER'S CHAPEL
Long before this solid, simple grey stone building was built on the edge of the land the Romans had constructed Othona fort to protect their settlements from the raiding Saxons. But eventually the Roman soldiers went home and the ordinary men and women of Essex became farmers. In AD 653 the Saxon king wanted to convert his people and he sent for St Cedd, who was to be a missionary. St Cedd built the chapel against the wall of the former fort, so it is also known as St Peter's on the Wall and a pilgrims' route – St Peter's Way – leads to it from inland. Services are still held here.

BRADWELL POWER STATION
This nuclear power station produced electricity from 1962 to 2002. It supplied over six million kilowatts of electricity each day – enough for the needs of several good sized towns put together. It was a focus for anti-nuclear activity, and on the day it closed (because it was no longer financially viable) – Easter Sunday 2002 – a number of Friends of the Earth were present to mark the occasion. Decommissioning the station involves de-fuelling both reactors, a process still being accomplished and likely to take several years.

Tiptree, Tollesbury and Layer Marney

20 miles

This is a brilliant ride. It takes you between rolling fields of crops to muddy, boat-filled creeks, across a modern reservoir full of birds and to the spectacular Tudor tower at Layer Marney. And it's one which provides you with good opportunities for cream teas at the beginning, the middle and the end. In fact, your starting and finishing point is the Tiptree Jam Shop, Tearoom and Museum.

Map: OS Landranger 168 Colchester, Halstead and Maldon.

Starting point: The Tiptree Jam Factory and Shop in Tiptree (GR 900156). Tiptree is about 10 miles south-west of Colchester, about 3 miles off the A12. The Jam Factory is at the southern end of the town on the B1023.

The Tiptree Tearoom is an ideal place for a snack (and a wander around the museum) before you go or when you return. There are various pubs en route and there is one in Tollesbury, which is your halfway point. Tollesbury also has a couple of places for coffee.

This ride gives you quite a comprehensive picture of this part of Essex and shows how varied it can be. There's nothing strenuous here, but be careful of the few miles you must travel along B roads.

Come out of the car park of the Jam Factory and **turn R** onto the B1023. **Turn R** after a few hundred yards, at the first turning you reach, towards Tolleshunt Major.

Follow this winding road for about 4 miles and **turn L** in Tolleshunt Major at the crossroads towards Tolleshunt D'Arcy. Continue for a mile and **turn R** off the road you are on for a few minutes in order to see the impressive pillared gateway of Beckingham Hall and its little church.

Turn round and go back and **turn R** onto the road you were on before, and then you can see the other side of the Hall. Continue into Tolleshunt D'Arcy. **Turn L** onto the B1026, pass the church and then

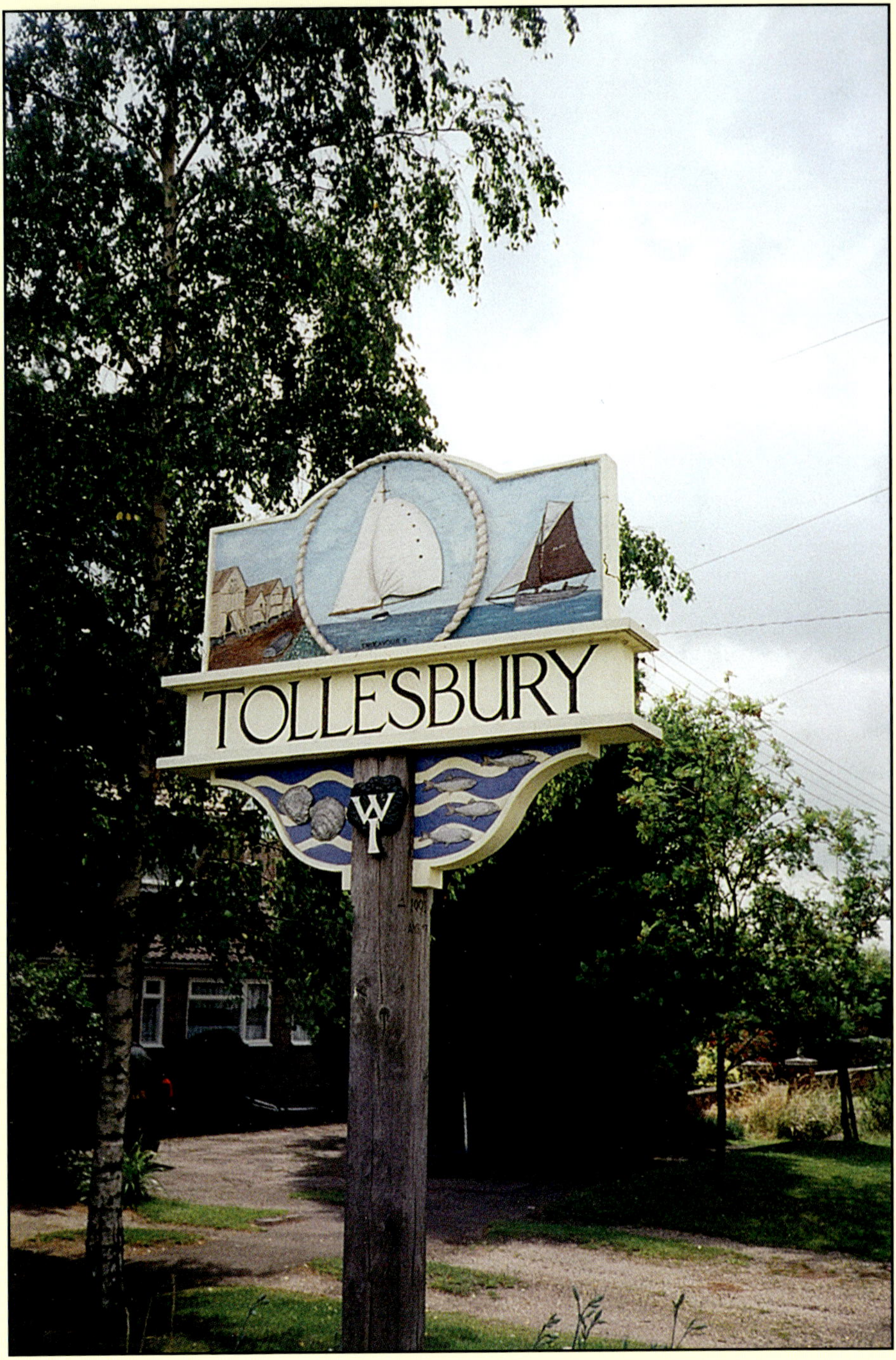

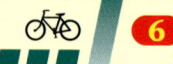

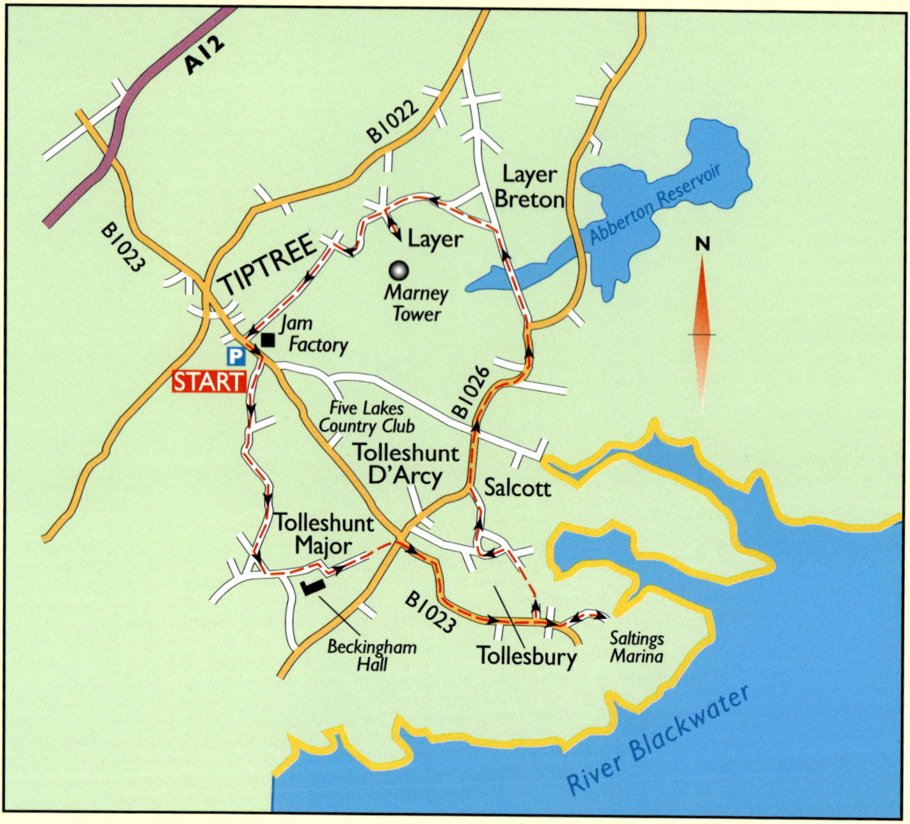

turn R at the Ristorant Piccolino and onto the B1023 towards Tollesbury.

Ride along here for about 4 miles and into Tollesbury. Look out for the attractive sign on your right. Go straight through, past the Hope and the King's Head, and, soon after the school, **bear L** at the fork, following signs to the industrial area and the waterfront. It looks an unlikely road but if you see plenty of boats in people's front gardens you are on the right track.

You pass a couple of cafés on your left. Keep on right down to the marina at Tollesbury Saltings, park your bike, and allow yourself an hour or so to watch the tides, boats and boat people.

Then ride back into and almost through Tollesbury and **turn R** by a former bank into North Road. Follow this road for about 2 miles and then **turn R** down Colchester Road, a small lane opposite Guisnes Court.

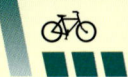

The road goes round a sharp bend to the left and then joins the B1026. **Turn R** onto this and then carry on past the Five Lakes Country Club on your left.

Soon after reaching Great Wigborough, **turn L** towards Layer and Colchester. After 1½ miles **turn L** towards Layer Breton and Birch.

This road takes you across the Abberton Reservoir. As you reach Layer Breton, **turn L** along a small lane, towards Layer Marney. **Turn L** again at a small junction and then **turn L** again at a small crossroads.

Follow this road down through Layer Marney and the tower is straight ahead. You can ride right up the drive to it.

When you have admired the tower go back down the drive, continue back along the road you were on and **turn L** down Woodview Road towards Rockingham's Farm. After a mile, when you reach a T-junction, **turn L** towards Tiptree.

Continue straight along here for 3 miles or so until you are back in Tiptree. **Turn L** into Chapel Road and then **turn L** at the crossroads. The Jam Factory is a few hundred yards further on.

● ●

TOLLESBURY
It is not too easy to distinguish between the land and the waters of Woodrolfe Creek. There are boats and bits of boats everywhere, mouldering hulks and modern hulls, and there's mud and marsh. Once over 70 fishing boats were moored in Tollesbury, and the wooden lofts where the sailmakers worked are still used. This is the perfect place for people to enjoy messing about in boats, or to watch others enjoy messing about in them.

The 'Crab and Winkle' railway line ran between Kelvedon, Tiptree and the quayside on the estuary here from 1904 to 1962, but in 1957 work was started on another major project across the Blackwater. This resulted in the giant chunky edifice of Bradwell Power Station, one of the first commercial nuclear generating stations in the UK, now being decommissioned.

ABBERTON RESERVOIR
The 6,000 million gallons of water here are pumped from the River Stour for the benefit of the people of Essex, but soon after its completion it was used by the RAF who wanted to practise their dam busting techniques in readiness for the subsequent bombing of German dams in 1942. Today, as the peaceful home for tens of thousands of water birds, it is enjoyed by hundreds of birdwatchers. Slow down as you ride and you are bound to see and hear something of interest.

LAYER MARNEY
As you follow this route towards Layer Marney you catch glimpses of an 80 ft many-windowed tower set amidst fields. This is your destination.

This impressive and elaborate gatehouse was the beginning of an unrealised dream. Unlike earlier gatehouses it was never intended as a defence, but rather as a statement of personal status and wealth. Henry, Lord

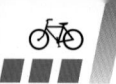 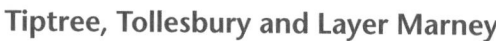
Marney was Captain of the King's Guard to Henry VIII, and he was a local man of Norman origins. But he died in 1523, when the main house – which clearly would have been an amazing building – had hardly been started. His vision would have been carried on by his son but he too died only two years later.

Even if you do not want to go inside, or if you arrive when the tower is shut, it's still worth riding down the drive to enjoy the splendid exterior.

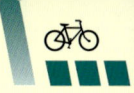

7

Canewdon and The Pagleshams

14 miles

This ride is within sight of suburbia and Southend, but it's a special one that takes you into a corner of Essex where there are muddy marinas, weatherboarded houses and open spaces. You won't find crowds because there are rivers to the north and south, and an almost empty island to the east. Prepare to be surprised.

Map: OS Landranger 178 Thames Estuary, Rochester and Southend-on-Sea.

Starting point: The Anchor pub at Canewdon (GR 901944) where parking is available for patrons. Please ask before leaving your car while you ride. Canewdon is about 6 miles north of Southend, which is on the A127.

You start at a pub and you find another one within 20 minutes, and then another in each of the Pagleshams. There's an extra one – the Shepherd and Dog – which you pass twice en route.

This route is compact and leads you to creekside dead ends (with some retracing of tracks). There are no hills but it is so flat that if there is a wind you will know about it.

Ride out of the Anchor and **turn L** immediately in order to see the beautifully restored church and the village lock up and stocks. Then turn back to the Anchor and ride from there along the main street past the shops.

After 1½ miles **bear L** along Creeksea Ferry Road and on across marshes. **Turn L** down the unmade lane to Creeksea Ferry Inn. Take your bike up onto the river wall behind it and look across the Crouch.

Ride along the grassy path sea wall and past the wharf and on to Essex Marina. Once on the tarmac surface past the Marina Bar and the end of the boatyard, turn away from the river here, out of the car park and along the small road that leads between an avenue of trees.

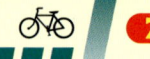
Creeksea Ferry

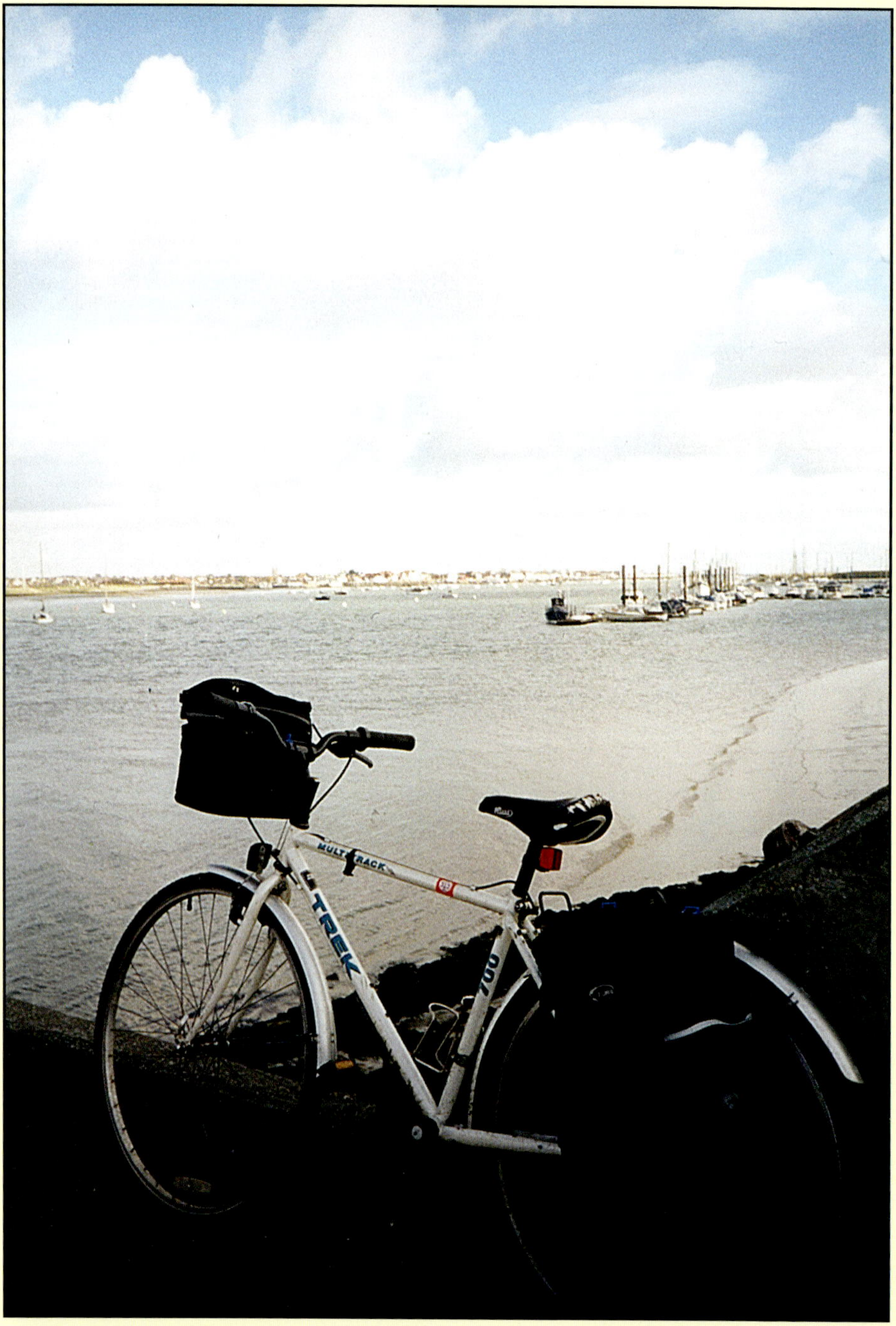

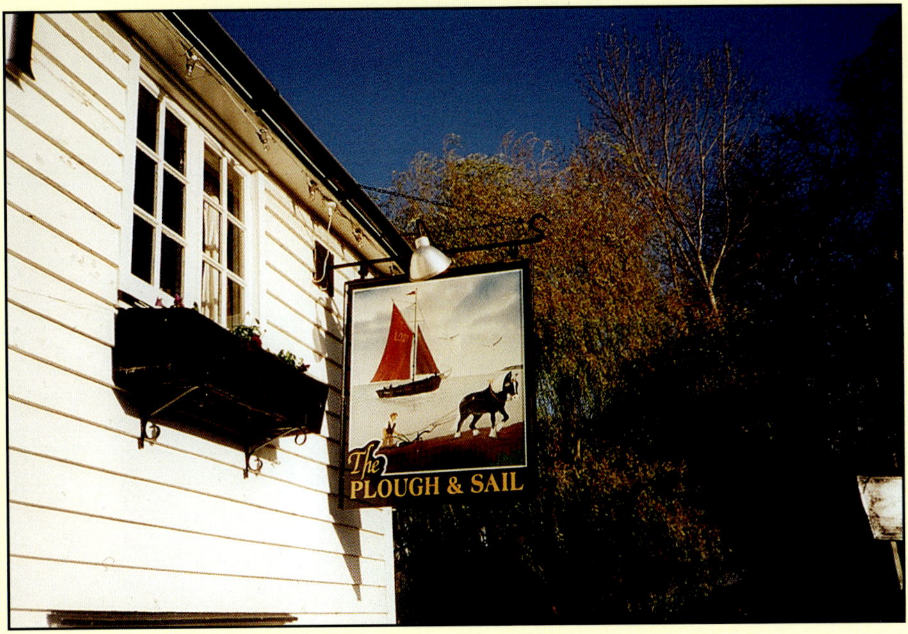

The pub at Paglesham Eastend

Follow the road as its turns to the right and continue along here for over 2 miles, past the entrance you took earlier to Creeksea Ferry Inn and ride back to a junction where you **turn L**, signposted to Rochford. You are still on Creeksea Ferry Road.

Carry on for a couple of miles and **turn L**. The Shepherd and Dog is to your right here. Ride straight along and stay on this road to Paglesham Eastend, ignoring (for now) the sign to Paglesham Churchend.

Just before you reach the Plough and Sail pub you'll see Cupola House on the left. If you want to see the boatyard and the rest of this tiny, unusual village, ride down the lane to the left of the pub.

Then **turn back** and return along the same road – there isn't another one. But **turn R** when you reach the sign for Paglesham Churchend and ride for a mile to the Punchbowl pub and another set of delightful weatherboarded houses.

Then **turn round** again and **turn R** back onto the road you were on. **Bear L** at the junction by the Shepherd and Dog which you saw earlier. It should be on your right as you ride past it.

Continue along here for a mile and then **turn R** towards Canewdon. Carry on for 2 miles and you come to a small crossroads in Canewdon. **Turn R** here and then **L** again, back to the Anchor pub which is on your left.

CANEWDON

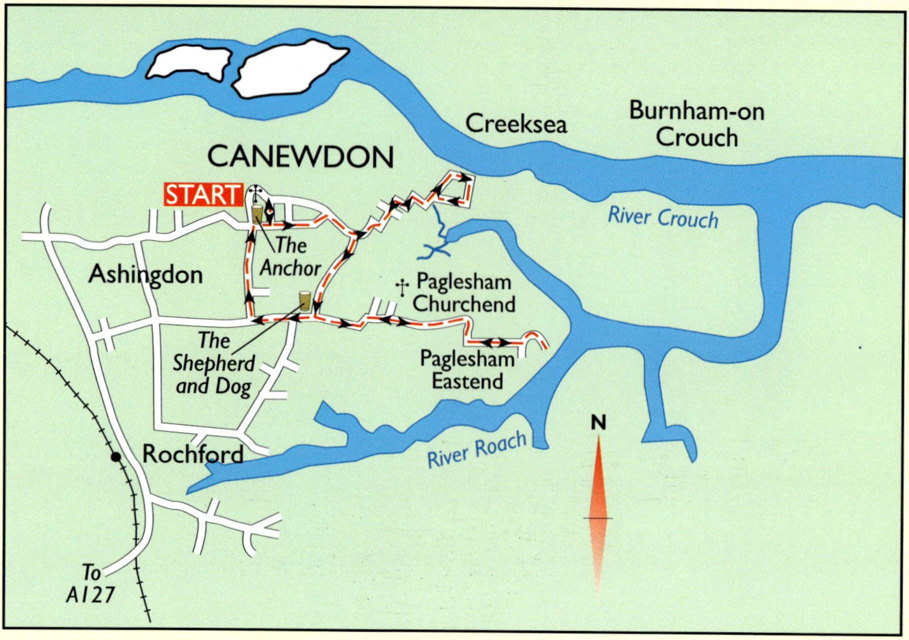

If you can arrange to climb up the tower of Canewdon church you will be rewarded with a panoramic view of this rivery part of Essex stretched out before you with Southend and then Kent visible to the south. In the Second World War and right up to 1973 there were other towers too: steel pylons erected as part of a Radar chain of defence.

There are also stories about Beacon Hill which was held by King Canute, the victorious Dane who launched his successful attack on the English monarch at nearby Ashingdon in 1016.

THE PAGLESHAMS

Although only a few miles apart, Paglesham Eastend and Paglesham Churchend are quite different in character. The latter is closer to the sea and its history is linked to boats, smuggling and oysters. Apparently Cupola House was built with money from smugglers' profits, and some of the walls in the garden have spaces in which contraband goods could be hidden. Paglesham Eastend is more pastoral, and it has some beautiful buildings.

North Fambridge, Cold Norton and Bicknacre

20 miles

This ride starts from the riverside, leads you along small lanes and through typical Essex landscapes of farms with grazing horses, cattle and sheep, and past woods and occasional fine houses. It then takes you back towards views of the muddy coastline and its distant sails. The placenames alone should pull you along on this ride: Cold Norton, Cock Clarks, Ilgar's Hall, Stow Maries.

There are one or two points on this route when you need to ride short distances on roads that are sometimes busy. There are also a few real hills. For these reasons this route is better for adults and is not recommended for children.

Maps: OS Landranger 168 Colchester, Halstead and Maldon and 167 Chelmsford, Harlow and Bishop's Stortford.

Starting point: The Ferryboat Inn, just south of North Fambridge (GR 852969). North Fambridge is 13 miles south-east of Chelmsford. Parking is available at the inn for patrons but please ask before leaving your car while you ride.

While the Ferryboat Inn is your start and finish point, there are other refreshment opportunities at the Fox and Hounds in Cock Clarks and, further on your way round, at pubs in Bicknacre and Stow Maries.

There are some hills.

From the pub car park **turn L** for a few hundred yards. You come to the very edge of the River Crouch. Then **turn round** and cycle back and straight out of North Fambridge. You pass the railway station on your right.

When you reach the junction with the B1012, **turn R** then **L** and carry straight on up Kit's Hill ahead on the B1010.

Turn L at the first turning along St Stephen's Road, and then **turn L** by the school.

Turn sharp R at the crossroads towards Purleigh. **Turn R** at the green and **R** again up Church Hill

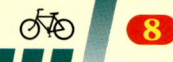

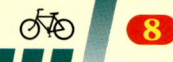

into the village to reach the church and the Bell pub. Then **turn round** and return to the green and go straight on up Mill Hill towards Cock Clarks.

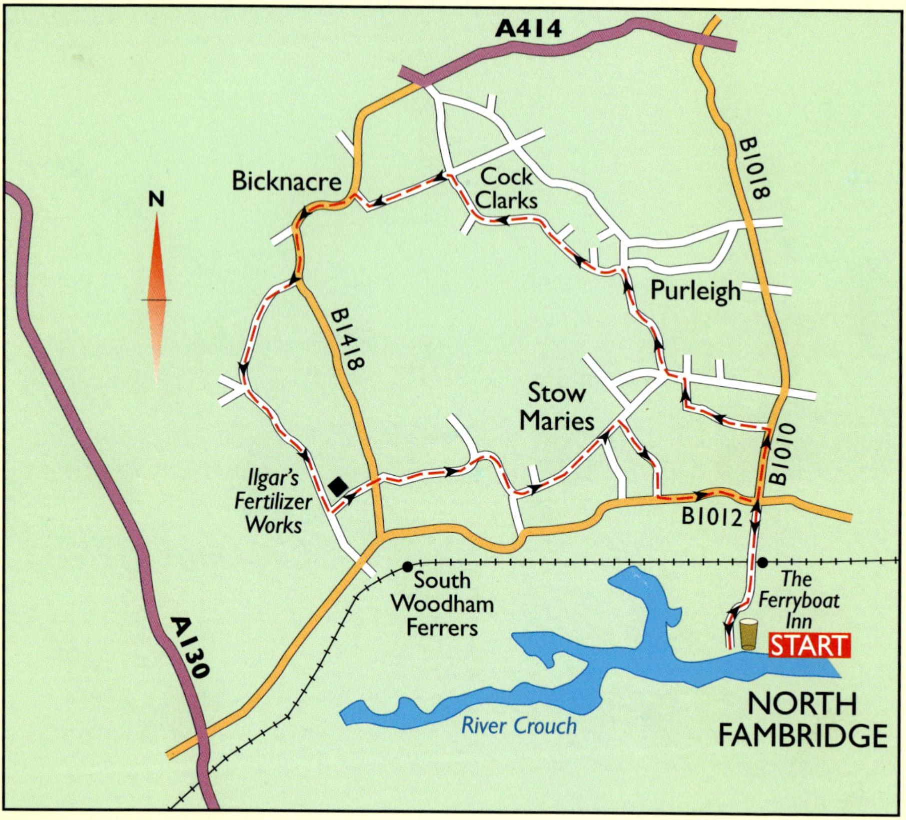

Pass the Fox and Hounds on your right, **bear R** and continue for a mile until you reach a crossroads. **Turn L** here along Slough Lane and then **L** at White Elm Road, the B1418.

Follow this into Bicknacre, **bearing L** at the White Swan and following signs to South Woodham Ferrers.

Just past the Brewers Arms **turn R** off this road onto Leighams Road, towards Hyde Hall Gardens.

After about 2 miles you reach a crossroads. **Turn L** here and then ride for another 2 or 3 miles until you see a pond on your left. **Turn L** here, by Ilgar's Fertilizer Works on the site of Ilgar's Hall.

Cross straight over the B1418 and onto a small lane. Ride along here until you pass Edwin's Hall. Ignore the turning to the left and follow the road you are on round a sharp bend to the **right** and, at the next junction, **turn L** towards Stow Maries.

Follow along here past the Prince of Wales. **Turn R** to see the church, and then return to the same road and then **turn R** into Honeypot Lane, just past a large house called Stow Bullocks.

Ride along here and down to the B1012. **Turn L** at the T-junction and ride for 2 miles until you are back at the junction you passed at the beginning of your ride. **Turn R** here and ride back into North Fambridge.

● ●

NORTH FAMBRIDGE

North Fambridge is separated from South Fambridge by the River Crouch, and a map shows roads that appear to lead straight into the water and indeed the high tide can flood the road. But there was once a ferry here – hence Ferry House and the 15th century Ferryboat Inn. It may not surprise you to know that smuggling used to take place here, but it was only in the 1980s that a yacht carrying cocaine moored not far from where the ferry used to run and armed police sealed the village off before arresting the smugglers. This excitement does not seem to have stopped the resident ghost at the Ferryboat Inn from continuing to move bottles about occasionally.

PURLEIGH

In 1897 Purleigh was chosen by a group of about 80 Russian exiles seeking somewhere to make a new community for themselves. They built their own homes and established a farming colony on the lane from Cold Norton to Cock Clarks. Freed from the Tsarist regime they were able to print Tolstoy's books and pamphlets and newspapers about their political beliefs. Despite the fact that some children went to the local school, most of them continued to speak Russian and to dress differently. However, the colony failed to thrive and within a few years they had gone.

Coggeshall, Cressing Temple and Stisted

17 miles

This ride starts in Coggeshall, a town with plenty of listed buildings and plenty of pubs. In Coggeshall is Paycocke's, an impressive heavily timbered house. As you ride out you pass Grange Barn, an outstanding centuries-old timber-framed building. Later you come to more magnificent barns at Cressing Temple. You should make time to visit at least one of these buildings, but if they are not open it is still worth looking at their exteriors. You will also pass through Silver End, an unusual village built in 1926.

The route is nearly all along quiet lanes and includes a stretch of public byway where you will probably be the only traveller. But note that you will have to cross the A120 twice and to go along it for about 100 yards.

Maps: Mostly OS Landranger 168 Colchester, Halstead and Maldon, but also 167 Chelmsford, Harlow and Bishop's Stortford.

Starting point: The Jubilee Clock Tower (GR 852227). This is in the centre of Coggeshall, which is off the A120, about 10 miles west of Colchester. There is a public car park nearby.

Coggeshall has a good choice of tearooms and pubs. En route you can buy refreshments at the Cressing Temple Barns, but these are not always open. There are pubs in Cressing and at Stisted, and Stisted also has a tearoom.

Because it's quite hilly, and you have to cross the A120, the ride is not a good one for children.

From the Jubilee Clock Tower ride down to the road on the far side of the little island with the street lights, and cross over to the White Hart pub. Leave the pub on your left and ride for a few yards and **turn L** into Bridge Street.

Ride across the bridge over the Blackwater and up Grange Hill. On your right is a sign to Grange Barn which is just off the road. It's worth having a look at the outside even if it is not open.

On the other, left-hand side of Grange Hill, opposite Grange Farm, is Abbey Lane which leads to the remains of an abbey and to a mill. **Turn L** down Abbey Lane if you

wish to see these.

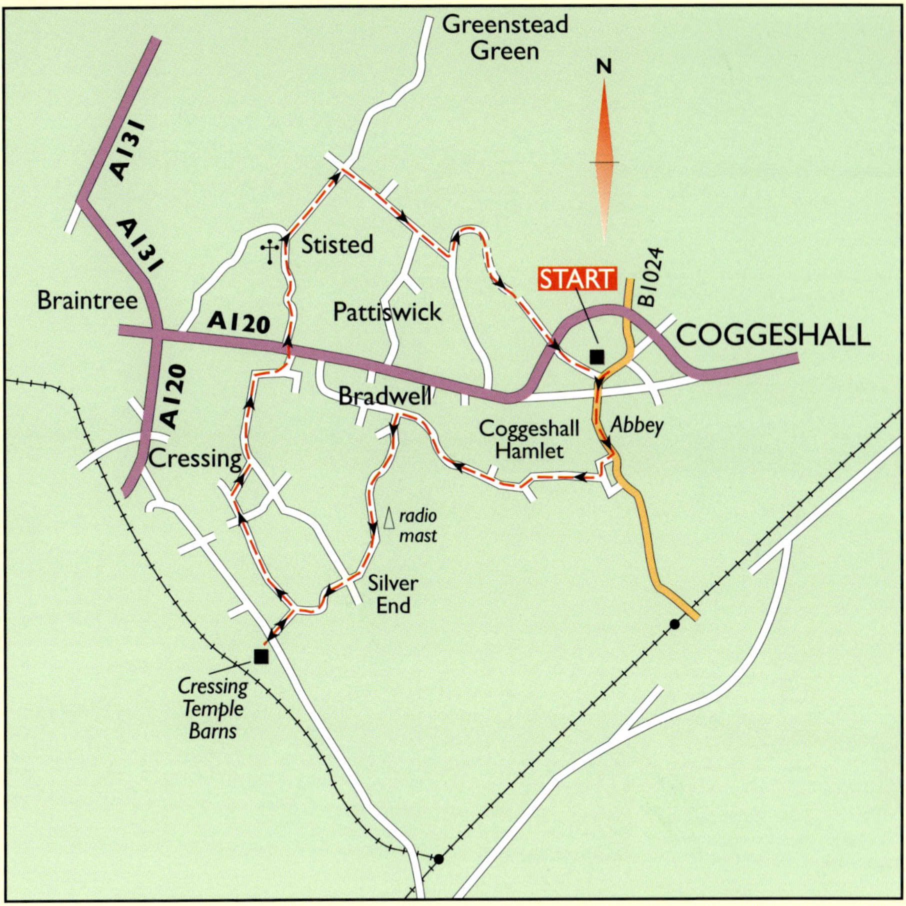

When you are back on Grange Hill carry on up the hill and **turn R** in Coggeshall Hamlet, onto an unsigned lane by a large white house called The Hamlet. **Turn R** at the next turning and ride for 3 or 4 miles between fields until you reach Bradwell church.

Turn L here towards Silver End and then **L** again. After 2 or 3 miles you pass a radio mast and enter the village by the modern Roman Catholic church. **Turn L** here, and then **R**, towards Cressing.

Keep L at the next junction, signed for Cressing Temple Barns. Follow the road down and just before you reach a main road **turn L** into the entrance to the Barns.

When you come out, **turn R** out of the entrance, up the way you came.

45

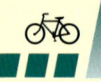
The Jubilee Clock Tower

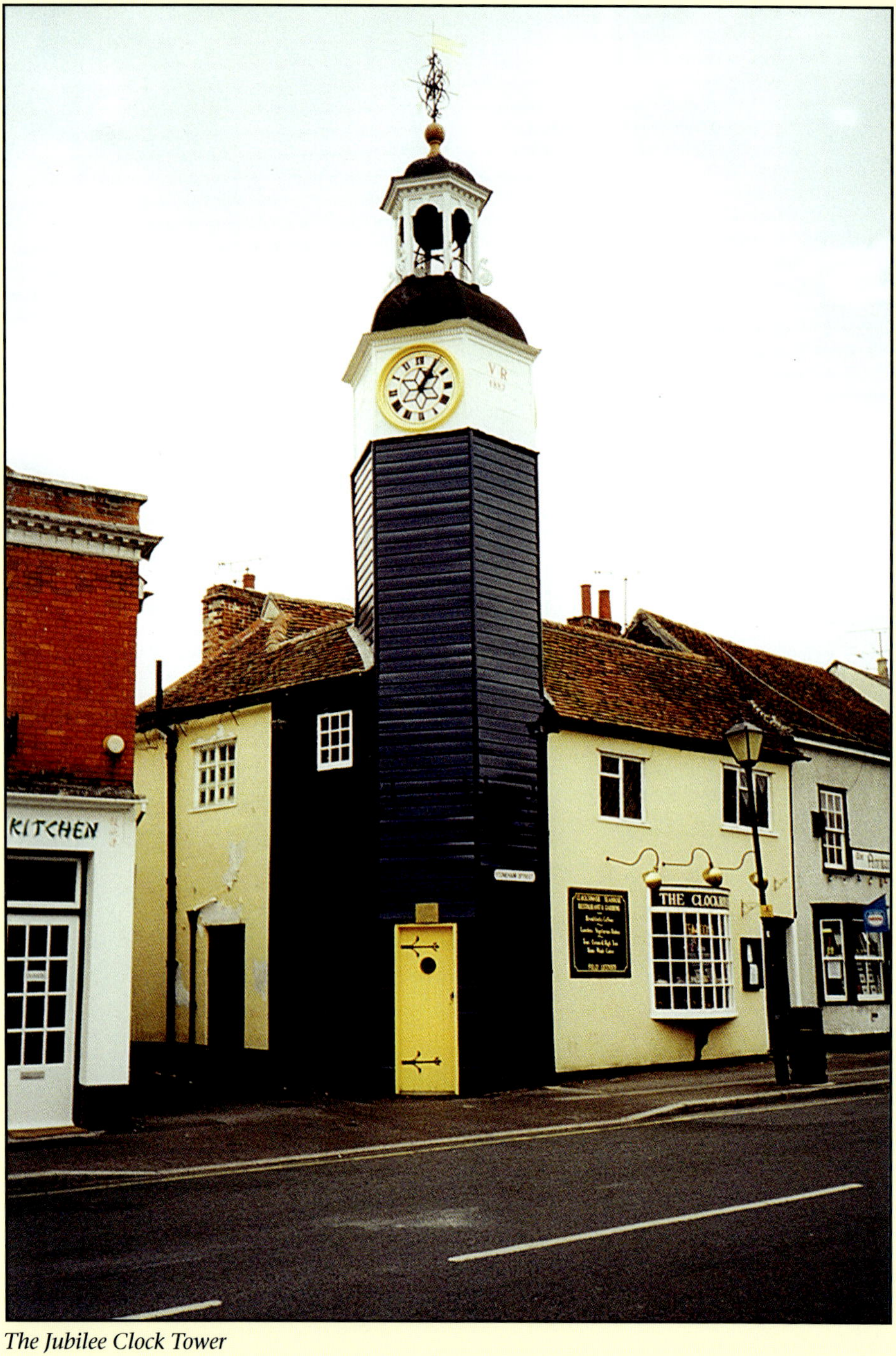

Then **turn L** towards Cressing. You pass Cressing church and the Willows pub. When you reach the fork in the road by the Three Ashes, **turn R** onto Lanham Green Road towards Stisted.

After 2 miles you reach the A120. Carefully cross over, **turn R**, and ride or walk about 100 yards and **turn L** off it towards Stisted.

Ride over the bridge and into the village, where it's worth making a small detour up the first road to your left towards Braintree. You'll find a tearoom and the Onley Arms. Carry straight through Stisted towards Greenstead Green. **Turn R** at the turning to Pattiswick, and then ride straight on, ignoring the next turning to Pattiswick.

Turn L at the junction, even though the sign says it is a dead end. After a few hundred yards **turn R** off your lane and onto a public byway. This is a wide but rather rough path that goes through woods and then fields for a couple of miles and takes you up to the A120.

Cross straight over and ride down the tiny lane opposite which takes you back into Coggeshall. If you wish to visit Paycocke's, ride straight down past the Jubilee Clock, past the White Hart and past

the turning to Bridge Street. It is on your left and well worth looking at.

• •

COGGESHALL

Coggeshall is built on land used by the Romans, and in the 1300s it had an abbey. This abbey is now in ruins, but its spectacular wooden tithe barn has been restored and is probably as strong now as it was 800 years ago.

The town has a wealth of attractive buildings, including the Jubilee Clock Tower and Paycocke's. Industry in Coggeshall was once centred on wool, but this was overtaken by lacemaking, and there is a display of exquisite lace in Paycocke's. But life was not all elegance here: in the 1840s a gang whose headquarters was a pub in Stoneham Street terrorised the local population until the police arrested the ringleaders as they tried to emigrate to America.

CRESSING TEMPLE BARNS

These amazing, huge barns were built on instructions from the Knights Templar, a fierce group of soldiers who served God and protected pilgrims travelling to the Holy Land in the 12th century. Cressing Temple was a farm 800 years ago and these barns date from between 1200 to 1700. Their size gives some indication of the amount of crops that were harvested and the huge scale of the farm.

Cressing Temple Barns house an exhibition and a tearoom, but they are not open all year round, so check if you wish to see more than the exterior.

Halstead and the Colne Valley

19 miles

This ride does not take you actually along the riverside, but rather along undulating lanes to the north and south of the Colne which is making its way to Colchester and the estuary. You'll be in or close to villages where the river was once an important feature: Earls Colne, White Colne, Wakes Colne, Colne Engaine. You start and finish the ride close by a fine watermill, and your halfway point is a bridge across the river.

This is a quiet landscape of meadows and woods, fields and hedgerows and most of the time you will meet few cars. However, the amazing viaduct at Chappel and Wakes Colne will remind you of the former importance of the railways.

Map: OS Landranger 168 Colchester, Halstead and Maldon.

Starting point: Chapel Street car park is off the main street near the post office (GR 813307). Halstead is on the A1124, 12 miles west of Colchester.

Halstead has an excellent range of places to eat. One of the most attractive is the Blacksmiths Tea Rooms by the river and Townsford Mill. Opportunities around halfway are at Greenstead Green Farm Shop and Café and the Swan at Chappel.

There are hills on this ride. Some you may wish to walk up; others you will not be able to resist zooming down.

Turn R as you exit from the car park onto the main street, and ride down this busy road for less than ½ mile, past Townsford Mill and round the bend.

Ride up the hill until you've passed all the houses on your left, and **turn L** into Oak Road. Follow this and bear left with the road you are on, and then **turn R**. Continue past a lake and Angling Club on your right, then **turn L** towards Greenstead Green. There's a farmshop and deli in the village. Cross over the small almost-crossroads into a little lane towards Burtons Green.

Keep straight on at the next junction (not turning towards Burtons Green).

The village pump

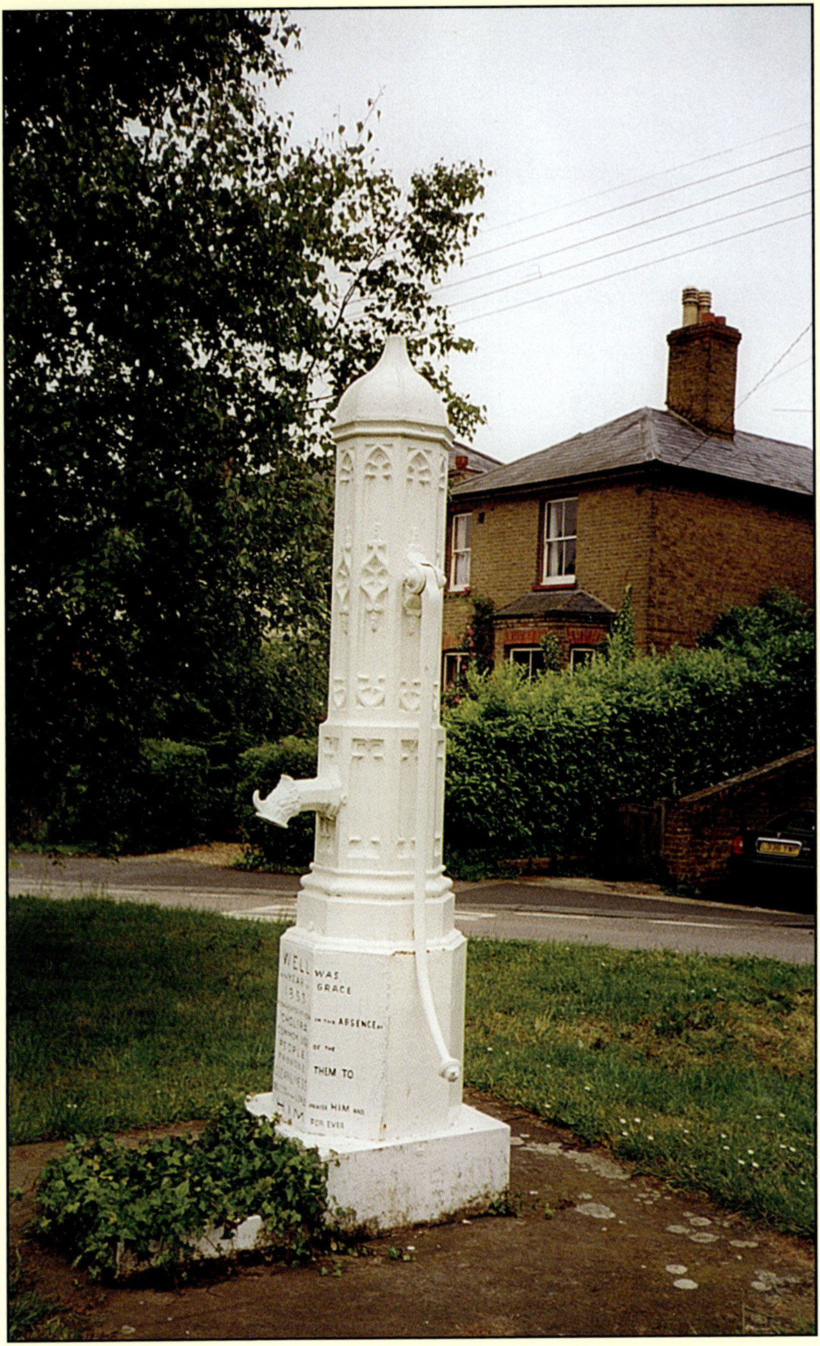

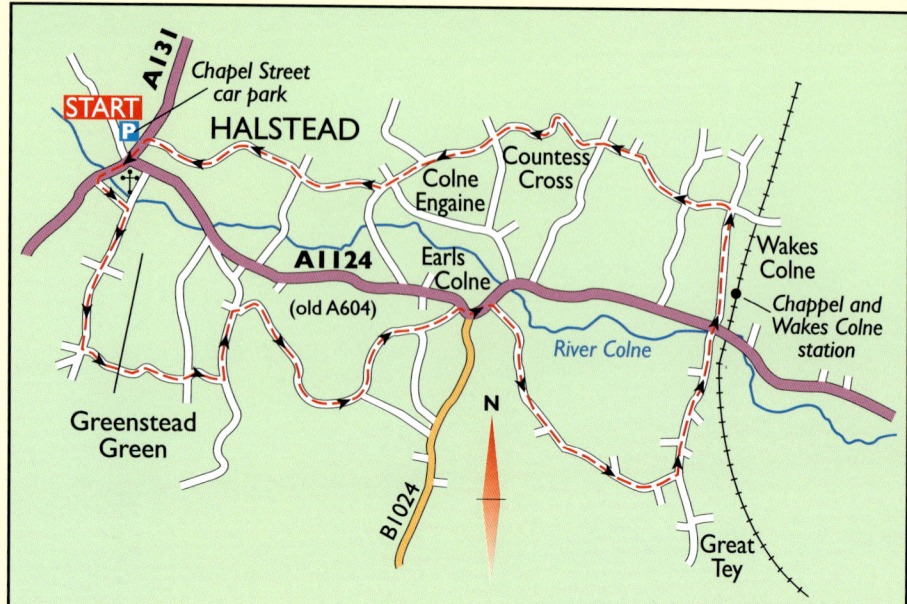

Then **L** at the next junction, on the road towards Earls Colne. Then **turn R** again (Stanstead Hall is on your left).

Turn R down a small lane towards Nightingale Hall. Follow this winding road round for a couple of miles until you see the airstrip ahead. **Turn L** onto Newhouse Road (on the left of the fence) and continue down into Earls Colne along Hayhouse Road. You'll pass the school, and come to the church on the corner at the A1124. **Turn R** here.

On your right, note the old pump with its interesting inscription. Ride along here and **turn R** onto Tey Road immediately after The Oxford House.

Keep on here for about 3 miles until you reach a T-junction. **Turn L** here, towards Chappel. Soon after you pass the sign stating that you are in Swan Street Chappel.

Continue down into Chappel and Wakes Colne and look out for the viaduct on your right. As you approach the crossroads with the A1124 you will see a little wooden-spired church on your left. Cross the river and find the Swan pub on your right.

At the main road go straight across on the road to Bures and to Chappel and Wakes Colne railway station. Ride up the hill for a mile or two to Wakes Colne Green, and **turn L** onto Lower Green, then very soon **R** onto Middle Green, and then **L** again onto Parkhurst Green Lane.

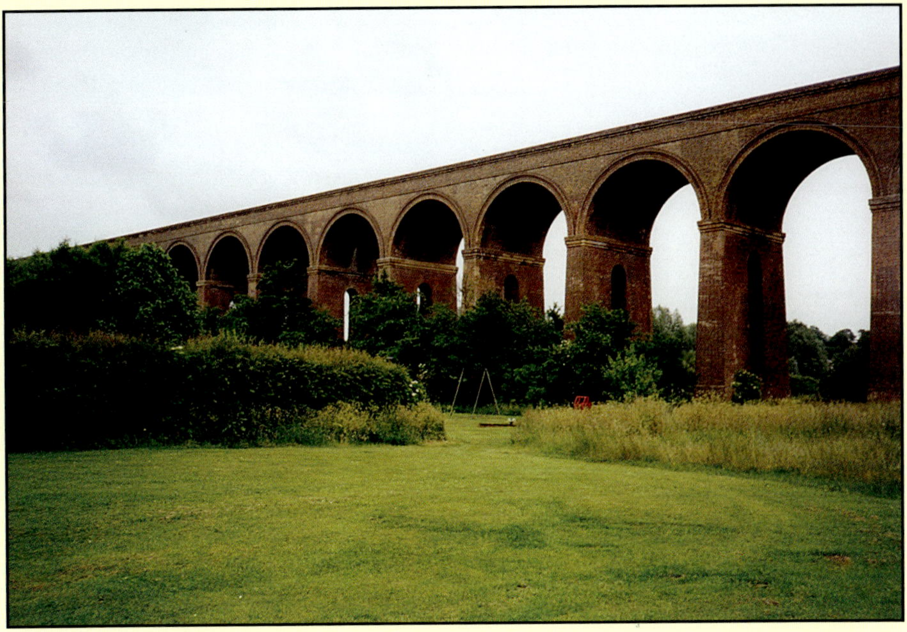

The Chappel and Wakes Colne viaduct

At the next minor crossroads go straight over towards Colne Engaine, marked for light traffic only. After a short distance, **turn L** again, still towards Colne Engaine. Follow this road for 1½ miles until you reach Countess Cross. **Turn R** and immediately **L** towards Colne Engaine and Halstead.

Follow the road you are on through Colne Engaine, and **turn R** at the church and then follow signs towards Halstead.

Ride for nearly 2 miles until you come to a T-junction on the edge of Halstead. **Turn R** towards The Maplesteads, past the cemetery on your left and the sports centre on your right. **Turn L** when you reach the A131 and follow the road down past the church and into the main street. Chappel Street is on the right.

HALSTEAD

In the 16th century Colchester became a destination for Protestants from the Netherlands fleeing from persecution. Before long some of them moved into Halstead where they worked as skilled, respected weavers of wool. Local jealousies led to them moving back to Colchester again, but Halstead workers ended up worse off as the excellent quality of the immigrants' work had enhanced their own. But nearly 300 years later Stephen Courtauld altered the watermill so that it could run looms, and his industry and workers thrived.

Now Townsford Mill houses antiques and collectables, so make sure that your bike has panniers.

CHAPPEL AND WAKES COLNE

These two villages are dominated by a spectacular 30-arch railway viaduct built in 1847 out of bricks made locally at Bures. It carried steam trains along the Colne Valley branch line from Marks Tey to beyond Sudbury and was originally planned to provide access to towns for rural communities. An important cargo that its builders could not have imagined was wagonloads of bombs for Second World War airfields. The line north of Sudbury was closed in 1962. The station for the two villages is located at Wakes

Colne where the East Anglian Railway Museum is housed and where enthusiasts have preserved a small section of line.

THE COLNE VALLEY

The length of the inland part of the Colne is only 32 miles. Its source is at Birdbrook near Haverhill and it flows through Halstead and the villages on this cycle route, down to Colchester (whose name it bears) and out past Wivenhoe, reaching the sea by Brightlingsea and Mersea Island. Although it once carried small craft as far inland as Halstead, the Colne was needed more for the power its water supplied to mills that ground corn or, as at Halstead, turned looms for clothmaking.

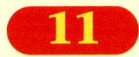

The Hedinghams, Little Maplestead and Wickham St Paul

18 miles

This ride takes you to the east and west of Castle and Sible Hedingham. The winding route is designed to protect you from main roads – though you will not avoid them completely – and to introduce you to a wealth of leafy lanes passing between fields that are richly green in summer and richly brown in autumn. Castle Hedingham, which is where you start and finish, has plenty for the curious pedestrian. There are several churches en route too, and their churchyards can be ideal places to pause, picnic and enjoy off-road peace.

This route takes you across main roads and, for a few hundred yards, along the A1124.

Maps: All but a small part of this route is covered by OS Landranger 155 Bury St Edmunds, Sudbury and Stowmarket. The rest is on 167 Chelmsford, Harlow and Bishop's Stortford and 168 Colchester, Halstead and Maldon.

Starting point: The crossroads at Nunnery Bridge, where Nunnery Road (on the north side of Castle Hedingham about five minutes ride from the castle) meets the A1017 (GR 775355). Castle Hedingham is about 18 miles north-west of Colchester. The town has few car parks (other than at the castle entrance where an entry charge for castle visits is made) but several pubs have car parks for patrons (please ask before leaving your car while you ride).

Castle Hedingham offers some choice about where to eat and drink, which will whet your appetite as you make your return journey, but there are other en-route opportunities. A particularly good place is Wickham St Paul, where you will find Spencer's Farm Shop and the Victory pub.

This ride takes you east and west rather than north and south, and it has quite a few twists and turns. It also has hills – none of which are too taxing. This route also includes a section of farm track.

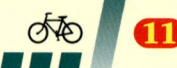

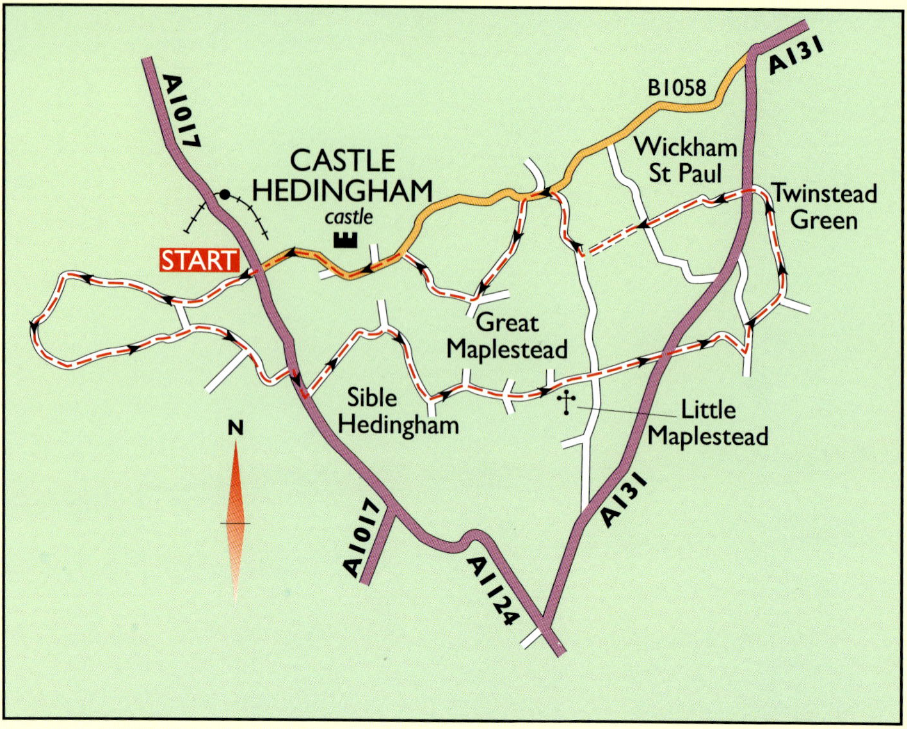

At Nunnery Bridge cross over the A1017 from Castle Hedingham (note the Cycle Repair sign as you go) and ride up the hill.

Turn R at the first junction towards Toppesfield. You'll pass the Bottle Hall pub on your right. **Turn next L** and ride along past Hillside Fishery and then Blois Hall.

Turn next L (signed to Blackmore End) and then **next L** again. Continue along here past Carters Barns and into Highstreet Green.

Turn R at the pump and follow the road down into Sible Hedingham. The church is on your left and, a little further on, the White Horse pub is on the right.

Turn R by the White Horse along Church Street, past the White Lion, and then **turn L** into Alexandra Road. When you meet the A1017 by a garage **turn R** and ride (or walk) for a few hundred yards and then **turn L** onto Alderford Mill Road by the town sign.

You first cross the young River Colne by a mill, and then the disused railway track. **Bear L** when the road forks, and then **turn R** at the road junction towards Great Maplestead.

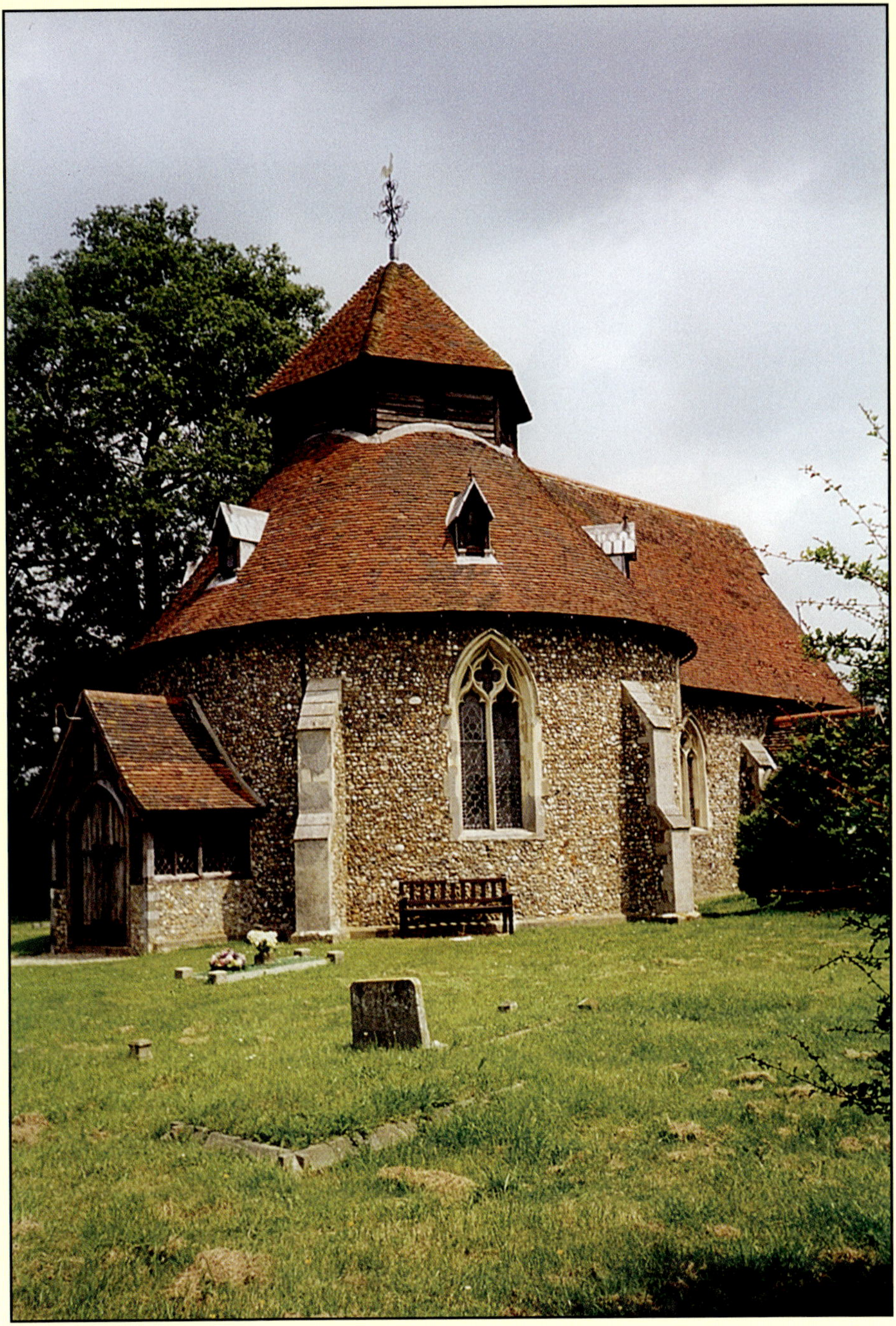

Little Maplestead church

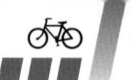

Then **turn L** towards Great Maplestead at a little triangle of grass by Lisley Cottage, and then **R** towards Little Maplestead at another little green by Barrett's Hall. Soon you see Maplestead Hall on your left and a small, unusual church on your right.

Turn L at the T-junction towards Gestingthorpe, and then **R** into Cock Road. You pass a water tower and then reach the A131 by a former pub, now called Little India. Cross over here and ride for a mile and a bit until you reach a small triangle at a junction.

Turn L here, and soon **R** and then **L** again by a big, black barn. This takes you to Twinstead Green. Ride on past the pump following the sign to Wickham St Paul.

Cross over the A131 again and continue until you reach a T-junction. **Turn L** if you want to go to Spencer's Farm Shop and café (it's only a few hundred yards). Otherwise **turn R** towards the attractive green at Wickham St. Paul. You'll see the Victory Inn (known as locally as the Ship) on your right. **Turn L** here, along a lane bearing the sign 'No Through Road'.

Ride across a concrete yard, following signs to the public footpath (do not turn left to Stones Farm). This is a wide grassy track which takes you between fields and down to a minor road where you **turn R**.

After a mile you reach the B1058. **Turn L** onto it and **turn L** off it after a few hundred yards. Continue for a couple of miles and then **turn R** at the first junction towards Castle Hedingham. Continue along here past Chelmshoe House Farm until you reach the B1058 again.

Turn L here and ride into Castle Hedingham. **Turn R** into Bayley Street, following signs to the castle. You may wish to visit this now or later, but to return to the starting point continue along Bayley Street and follow straight on into Nunnery Street.

• •

CASTLE HEDINGHAM
This ancient and interesting little town should be explored on foot. Set in open grassland the castle is an impressive example of a square Norman keep which contains a barracks, cellars and a magnificent banqueting hall. If you don't have enough time to visit it, a walk through the small streets and squares will provide you with occasional glimpses. The castle was built by the de Vere family, who also built the church. Falcons were once kept in the Falcon Inn, and 150 years ago the Bell was busy as the posting house used by stage coaches en route from Bury St Edmunds to London.

LITTLE MAPLESTEAD

It is a surprise to find this church well off the beaten track. It is one of only four round churches in England, and was built by the Knights Hospitallers of St John, the oldest order of Christian chivalry. The first knights defended pilgrim routes to Jerusalem – where the church is round – and there are still about 8,000 knights today. Annually, on St John the Baptist Day, there is a service in Little Maplestead for the leaders of the Order dressed in their regalia, followed by a procession that includes members of the St John's Ambulance Brigade.

WICKHAM ST PAUL

Ten centuries ago this village was connected with the Dean and Chapter of the cathedral dedicated to another saint – St Paul. Like numerous other villages in farming areas it once had its own shop, tradesmen, local employment on the land, school and even a youth club in the 1950s. On hot days tired cyclists have two choices for refreshment. They can either go to the Spencer's Farm café or to the pub, and perhaps stretch out for a snooze under one of the huge trees on the beautiful green. Or maybe both!

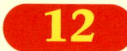

The Hanningfield Reservoir and Stock

12 miles

This is a reservoir ride – you start and finish right by the wide reservoir and your route gives you views across it at some places although at others it is hidden. You also make a detour into the village of Stock. It's really a place for fishing and even if you don't take or hire a rod you will be able to buy trout at the Fishing Lodge.

Map: OS Landranger 167 Chelmsford, Harlow and Bishop's Stortford.

Starting point: Hanningfield Fishing Lodge at South Hanningfield (GR 737977). South Hanningfield is about 8 miles south of Chelmsford, a few miles west of the A130.

The Fishing Lodge has a café restaurant overlooking the reservoir. There are several pubs (and a fish and chip shop) in Stock, including the Bear and the Cock, another at West Hanningfield and another almost at the end of the route. It might be a good idea to take a picnic and explore a path off the route to discover your own private picnic place by the water. And it's a ride where you can't help enjoying the arches of trees over the roads.

This is a steady, short and easy route with no hills.

Ride out of the car park, up to the road and **turn R**. After a mile **turn R** again onto Hawkswood Road.

Follow this road for several miles and then ride across the end of the reservoir. **Turn R** on to Downham Road opposite Whitelilies Farm, towards Stock.

Turn L up Mill Road and into Stock. You will come to the Bear and, on the other side of the B1007, the Cock. **Turn L** and ride for a ½ mile or so if you wish to see the very unusual flint church with its wooden belfry. When you are ready **turn round** and ride back out of Stock and along Mill Road but **turn L** onto Mill Lane and ride past the old tower windmill.

At the T-junction **turn L** and then **turn R** towards West Hanningfield. Ride along here for 2 or 3 miles until you reach a junction by the Three Compasses on your right. **Turn R** here and continue straight along the road to visit the church on your left.

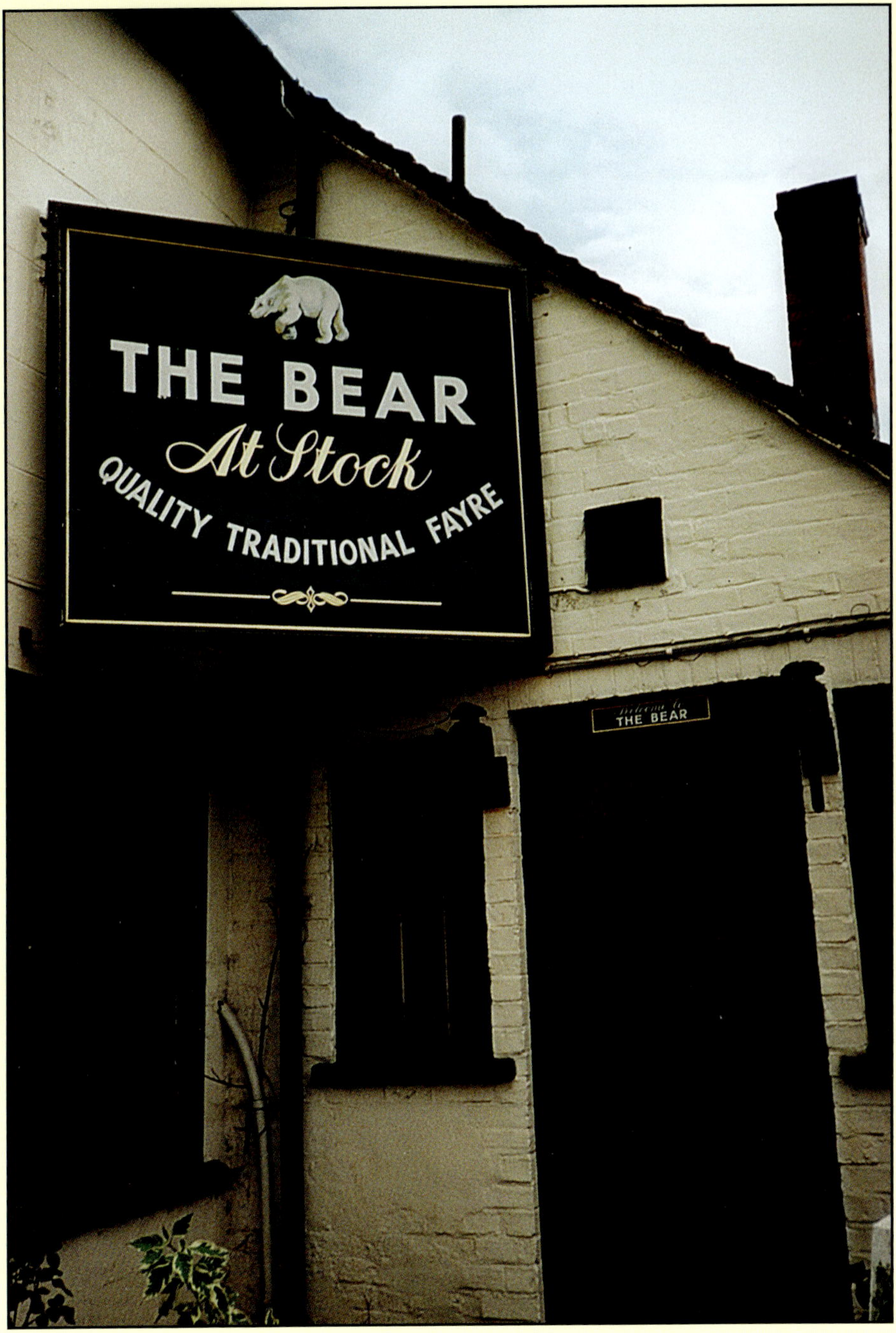

One of the pubs on the route

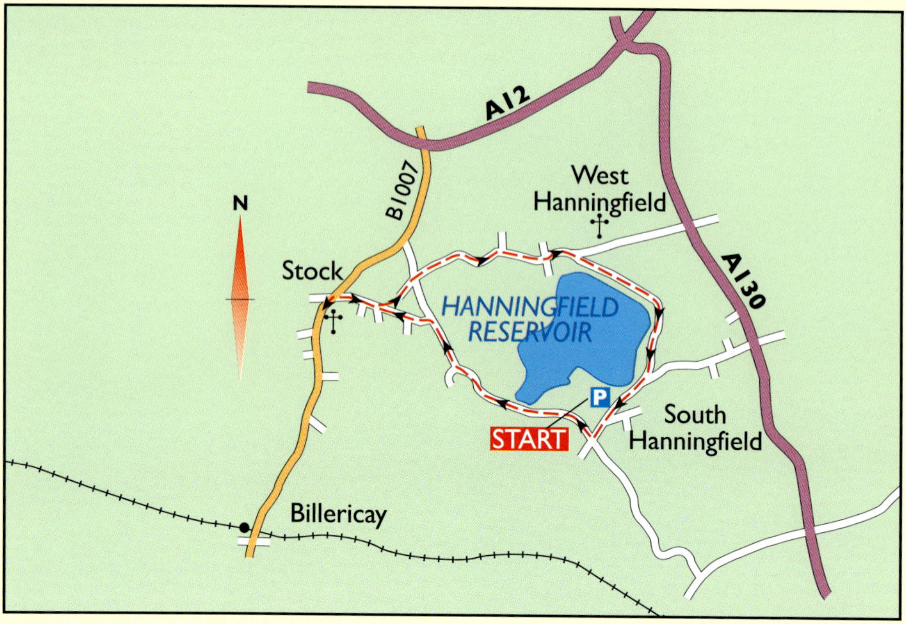

Then **turn round** and ride back and **turn L** on to Middlemead, a road signposted to the reservoir. Ride along here, parallel to the reservoir though you will lose sight of it and not see it for a couple of miles.

Just carry straight on and **turn R** at the T-junction, following signs to the reservoir. You pass the Old Windmill pub just before you **turn R** down to the Fishing Lodge.

• •

HANNINGFIELD RESERVOIR
This was started in 1950 and completed by 1957. It occupies a shallow (maximum depth about 51 ft) natural dip in the land that used to be farmland. The remains of a few houses lie under the water – notably Fremells, the once fine home of the family of John de Hemande, and Pynning's Farm and cottages.

Now the reservoir is a trout fishery with a shop devoted to the needs of people who fish. Even if the only fish you see there are dead ones in cases or in fridges, you are bound to see plenty of live water birds.

STOCK
Stock was settled by the Saxons and its name is derived from Herwardstoc, which may refer to the ownership of the land by the steward or lord who had cleared the land of stocks (or tree stumps). The name later turned into Stock Harvard, and now it's just Stock. Its wooden church – especially the belfry – is famous and in 1940 it withstood the explosion of landmines in the churchyard.

Richard Twedye was buried in the churchyard in 1574. He was a soldier who had almshouses built for 'foure poore knights' and they are still there on the green opposite the church.

13
The Belchamps, Pentlow and Foxearth

13 miles

This ride takes you in a rough circle in the soft rolling agricultural land of north Essex. For almost half the time you'll be close to the River Stour which is the border with Suffolk, although it's sometimes quite hidden and you won't see it until you find yourself on a little bridge. You'll pass handsome houses and peaceful churches. There's a particularly lovely church in Belchamp Walter.

If you had been here a hundred years ago the farm workers and farm animals would have been all around you. Now it is possible to cycle between these vast fields of cereals and sugar beet and hardly see anyone at work except the drivers of huge combines and tractors.

Map: OS Landranger 155 Bury St Edmunds, Sudbury and Stowmarket.

Starting point: The car park at Rodbridge Picnic Site (GR 857437). This is on the B1064 a couple of miles to the south of Long Melford and the same distance to the north of Sudbury. Sudbury is on the A134 about 15 miles south of Bury St Edmunds.

There is only one place for refreshment actually on the route – the Half Moon in Belchamp St Paul – but a small detour over the Stour into Cavendish will take you to two pubs by a pretty village green.

This route is entirely along quiet, rural roads. In fact, many of them could be called lanes.

Come out of the car park and **turn L** over the bridge and into Essex. **Turn L** immediately up a lane, pass Borley village hall and ride up to the church. It's worth a look back here at the view. There's a flint wall opposite and there used to be a rectory behind it – supposedly the most haunted house in England.

Turn L at the crossroads, towards The Belchamps. **Turn R** at the T-junction, and continue past Eyston Hall. Cross the bridge over Belchamp Brook, and head on towards Belchamp Walter. Then **turn L**, following signs to the church and hall. At a small green with a letterbox **turn L** again. Go down what seems like a secret little lane past Munt House and continue until you reach the church on your left and the hall on your right.

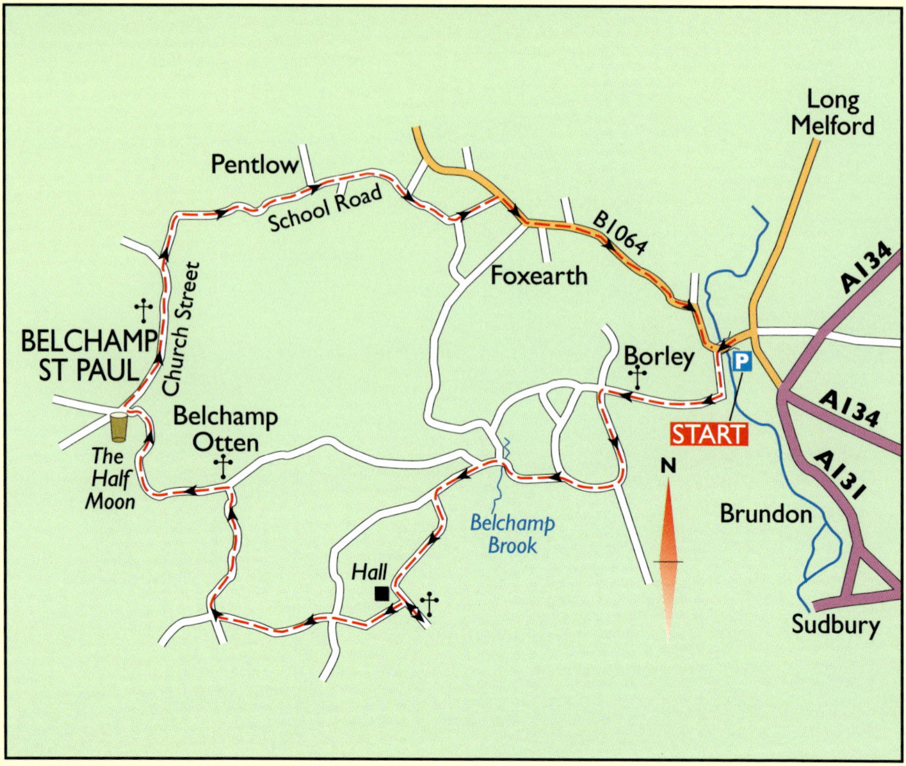

Long Melford

Pentlow

School Road

B1064

A134

Foxearth

BELCHAMP ST PAUL

Church Street

Borley

P

A134

Belchamp Otten

START

A131

The Half Moon

N

Brundon

Belchamp Brook

Hall

Sudbury

After you've visited the church, return to the green with the letterbox and **turn L** towards Belchamp Walter. Note the tall ruin on your left as you ride straight through Belchamp Walter. Cross straight over the crossroads by the pond. **Turn R** at the T-junction towards Belchamp Otten and follow the road round.

In Belchamp Otten, **turn L** at the T-junction towards Belchamp St Paul, ride past the church and **turn R** (again towards Belchamp St Paul). When you reach the T-junction, **turn L** for the pretty green and the Half Moon pub. Then ride back the way you came (but

don't turn back up Otten Road where you came from) and continue up the road you are on and past the church which is on your left.

Soon **turn R** towards Pentlow; and, once in Pentlow, follow the sign to Foxearth. Look out for Bull's Tower in the woods on your left. You can see it more clearly from a little further on by the big gates to the hall. Join the B1064, **turning R** towards Foxearth, and when you are there **turn L** at what looks like a T-junction, towards Long Melford. The old school is on your left.

Follow the B1064 for a couple of miles

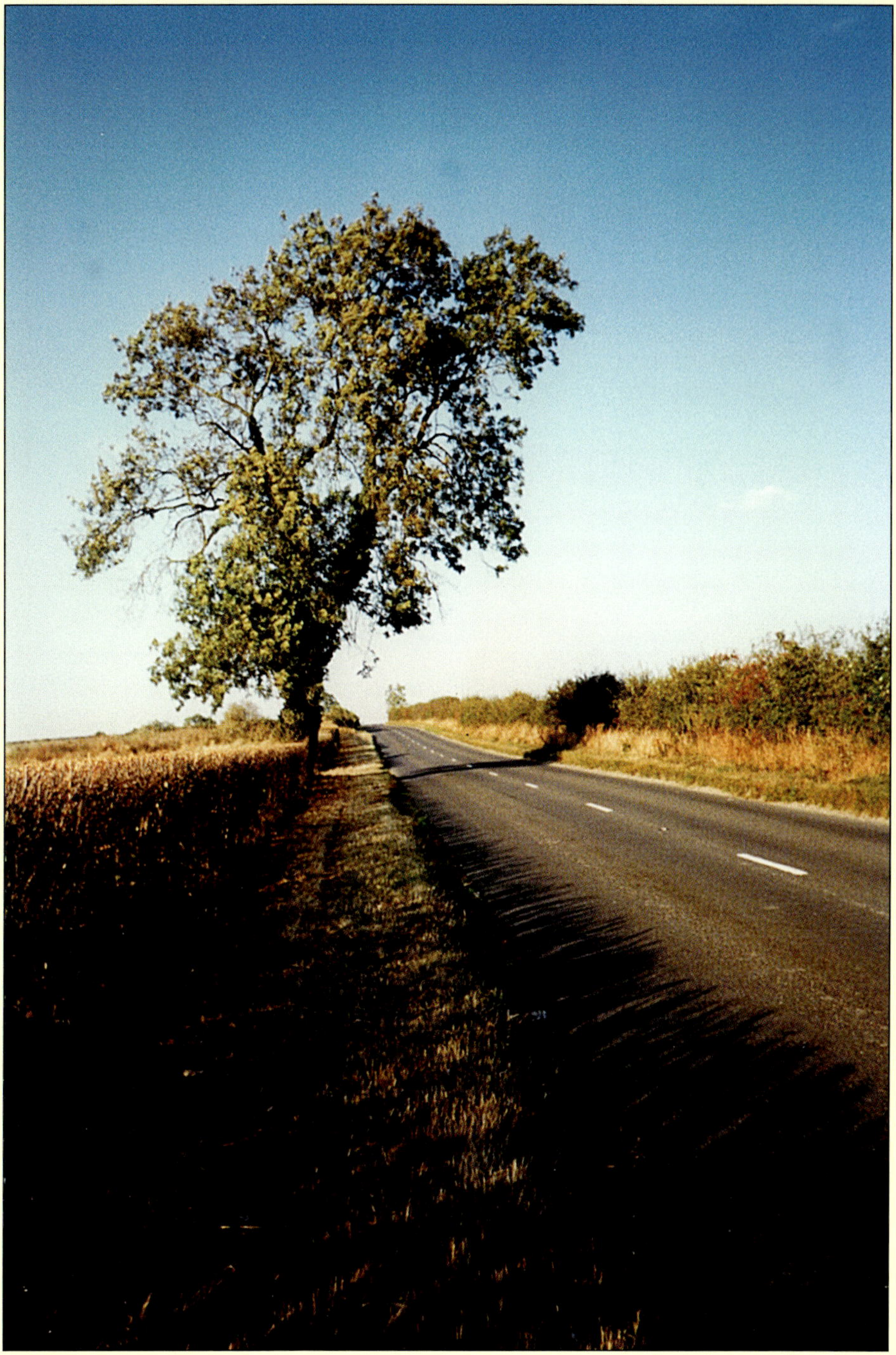

then **bear L** and so ride back across the bridge by Rodbridge Picnic Site.

. . . .

BULL'S TOWER, PENTLOW

This octagonal tower was built in 1859 by the Reverend Bull in the garden of his rectory in memory of his parents. Having no actual function, it is a true folly. Here's a transcript of the entry about it in the edition of *The Builder* of 18th June 1859:

The tower is octagon [sic] 90 feet in height, of the Tudor style of architecture, embattled, and built of red bricks, and variegated with designs in black. On the top is a flag staff. The summit is reached by a spiral oak staircase, of 114 steps, lighted by windows placed in the sides of the tower.

From the top a view is obtained, embracing forty one churches, sixty windmills, two castles and several large halls and estates. The tower, according to printed statements, was designed and erected by Mr L. Webb of Sudbury, superintended by Mr. J Johnson, architect, of Bury St Edmunds.

Unfortunately the tower is in private hands, so you'll have to imagine climbing the 114 steps and guessing where all those windmills once stood.

THE RIVER STOUR

The Romans probably used the Stour for trade and transport from the river's estuary at Manningtree right up to Long Melford. By 1705 it must have fallen into disrepair because an Act was passed to make the river navigable.

The main vessel on the Stour for the carriage of goods was 'the lighter', measuring 47 ft long by nearly 11 ft wide. They could carry a weight of up to 13 tons. Lighters were built from timber at several dry docks in Flatford and in 1815 Constable painted a picture entitled *Boat building near Flatford Mill*. The lighters were towed in pairs by horses between Sudbury and Brantham tidal lock, a distance of nearly 24 miles. From Brantham they could be floated on the tide to Mistley Quay. The main goods carried on the Stour were coal, corn and bricks. Coal was moved upriver, corn and bricks in the opposite direction.

Now there are far fewer locks than there once were, but the river is still enjoyed by many people in small craft.

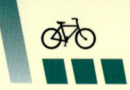

Felsted and The Easters

18 miles

This ride takes you in a deep sweep through a swathe of Essex farmland: for much of the way you'll have views. Starting from Felsted, which gives its name to a traditional public school, you'll pass a former brewery sited next to the River Chelmer, which is flowing slowly to and through Chelmsford, and you'll go through Good Easter where a small hoard of Roman coins was found using metal detectors. The hoard was declared treasure trove in 1998.

Map: OS Landranger 167 Chelmsford, Harlow and Bishop's Stortford.

Starting point: The car park by Felsted church (GR 677204). Felsted is about 9 miles north of Chelmsford.

Felsted has two pubs and a restaurant. There are other pubs in Pleshey and Good Easter, and in High Easter, which is just past the halfway mark. There are plenty of places en route where you could sit and snack for ten minutes, enjoying the view.

You'll probably notice ups and downs on this ride, especially if it's windy – but there's nothing too strenuous.

Ride out of the car park, **turn L** and then immediately **R** along Chelmsford Road, the B1417. Ride through Causeway End and on for about 3 miles until you reach the now closed down Hartford End Brewery on your right.

Go straight on over the bridge and on for a mile until there is a road marked 'No Entry' on your right. **Turn R** here, and push or scoot your bike along it to the A130. Cross over here carefully and ride for a few hundred yards and then **turn L** towards Pleshey.

Follow along here and **turn L** at a small T-junction. Ride on for 2 more miles until you join another road leading into Pleshey. Ride up the hill past the Leather Bottle. There's a sign to the castle on the left but you cannot get near the ruins.

Continue up the hill past the White Horse, past the church on your left and on to a T-junction where you **turn L**. Ride on for 1½ miles on a road signposted towards Mashbury and The Chignals.

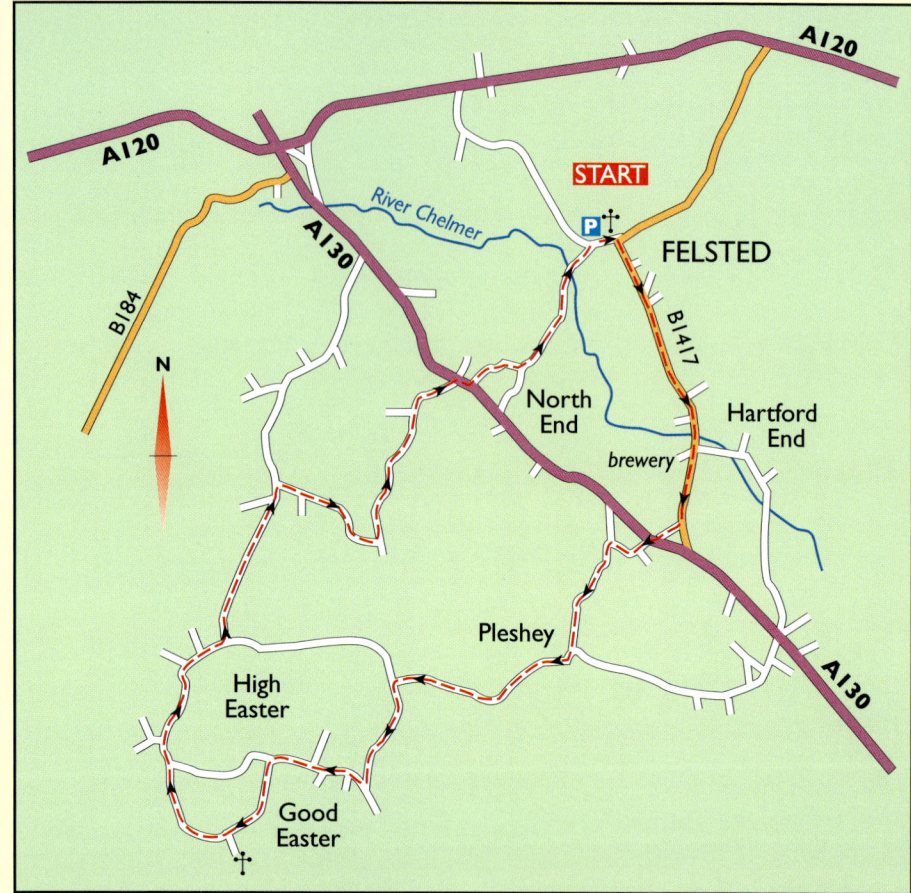

Turn **R** onto a minor road signed to Good Easter. After another couple of miles **bear L** towards Good Easter. Ride straight through Good Easter, and then **turn L** at the T-junction for a hundred yards or so in order to see the church with its wooden steeple. Then **turn round**, and ride past the turning you came from and straight on towards High Easter.

Keep going along here for several miles until you reach High Easter.

Ride past Punch Bowl, and **turn sharp R** with the road you are on, and take the **first** L, signposted towards Barnston.

Ride up here for 2 more miles and then, soon after you pass the water tower on your right, **turn R** and follow this lane along for about 3 miles and you reach the A130 again.

Turn R onto it and then turn **immediately L** towards North End.

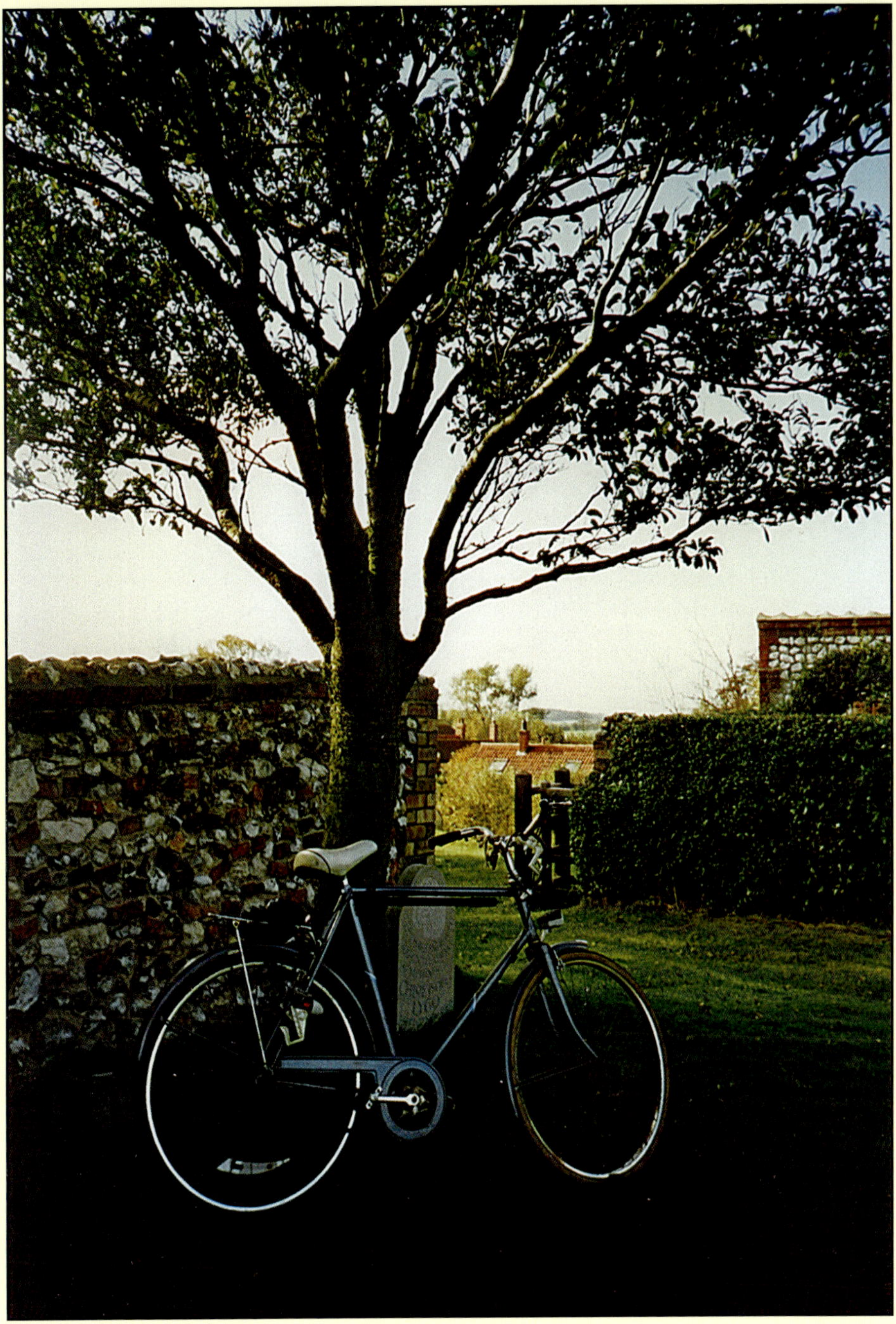

A shady spot to rest awhile

Turn **L** in North End towards Felsted and continue for the final few miles back, past a watermill, to Felsted.

• •

FELSTED

In 1564 a local nobleman, Lord Rich, who was Lord Chancellor, founded Felsted School for boys born on his manors and farms. He is buried in a tomb with a sumptuous marble memorial in Felsted church. On the outside of a substantial timber-frame house that faces the church is an inscription 'Geo. Boote made this: 1596'. The nearby Guildhall – which was where Lord Rich first opened Felsted School – was built even earlier. Under the arch of the former Guildhall is the 'herring window'. This window, which depicts a barrel encircled by fish, was made because Lord Rich made an endowment of barrels of herrings and kippers for the poor of Felsted.

The school is now co-educational and must be very different from when Oliver Cromwell – who married a local girl – sent his four sons there.

GOOD EASTER

The name of this village has nothing to do with lots of Easter eggs. The word 'Easter' is derived from the Old English 'eowestras' which meant sheepfolds, and 'Good' may come from Lady Godiva, a local noblewoman.

In 1885 Good Easter's church steeple was seen to be on fire. A man set off on horseback to Chelmsford (7 miles away) to fetch the two fire brigades that were based there. Meanwhile, back in Good Easter, men were trying to save the pews, organ and other wooden furniture. One of the horse-drawn fire brigades started out immediately, but the other one, which set out later, gave up when they realised that they would not get all of the insurance money. It took some hours to extinguish the fire but within a year the severely burned church was repaired.

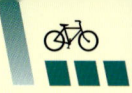

15

Thaxted, Finchingfield and The Bardfields

14 miles

This gem of a ride takes you through stunning villages, past a handful of unique churches and it gives you wide views over peaceful expanses of countryside. As it's in the most attractive and popular part of Essex it would be sensible not to do this route at the busiest weekends in summer.

Thaxted and Finchingfield are almost textbook examples of the traditional English village, but enjoy whatever you find in between them – a field of blue linseed, a windmill, or a tractor which won't let you – or you can't – overtake. The substantial houses were built and occupied by people with substantial wealth, and they still are. This bike ride will enrich you too.

Maps: OS Landranger 167 Chelmsford, Harlow and Bishop's Stortford and a tiny bit of 154 Cambridge and Newmarket, Saffron Waldon.

Starting point: Thaxted church (GR 610310). Thaxted is on the B184 about 17 miles north of Chelmsford. There are at least two car parks in Thaxted.

This ride is peppered with places to eat and drink. You have plenty of choice for pubs and tearooms, particularly in Thaxted and Finchingfield.

Be prepared for some quite steep hills.

Face up away from Thaxted church and the Swan pub and ride along Newbiggen Street. **Turn R** onto the B1051 towards Great Sampford when you reach the Thaxted Hall Woodlarks Restaurant on your right.

Continue for 4 miles and then **turn R** onto a minor road signposted to Little Sampford. After 2 or 3 miles you reach a junction by Little Sampford Hall. On the far side of the junction is an exquisite little church.

Turn L here towards Little Sampford and Finchingfield. Ride down the hill and across a bridge and **turn R** towards Finchingfield.

Ride up a longish hill and then down into Finchingfield which is

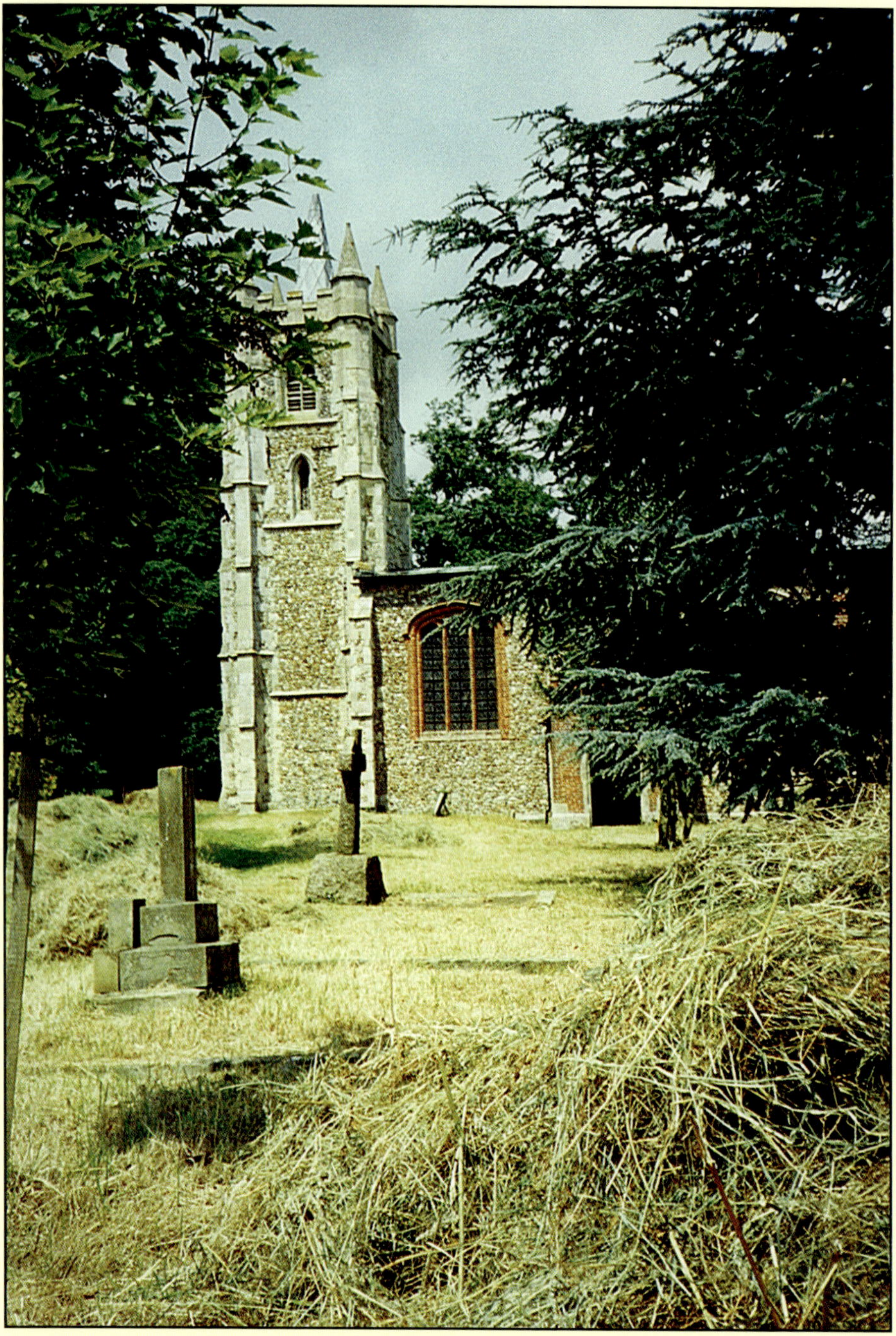

Little Sampford church

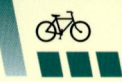

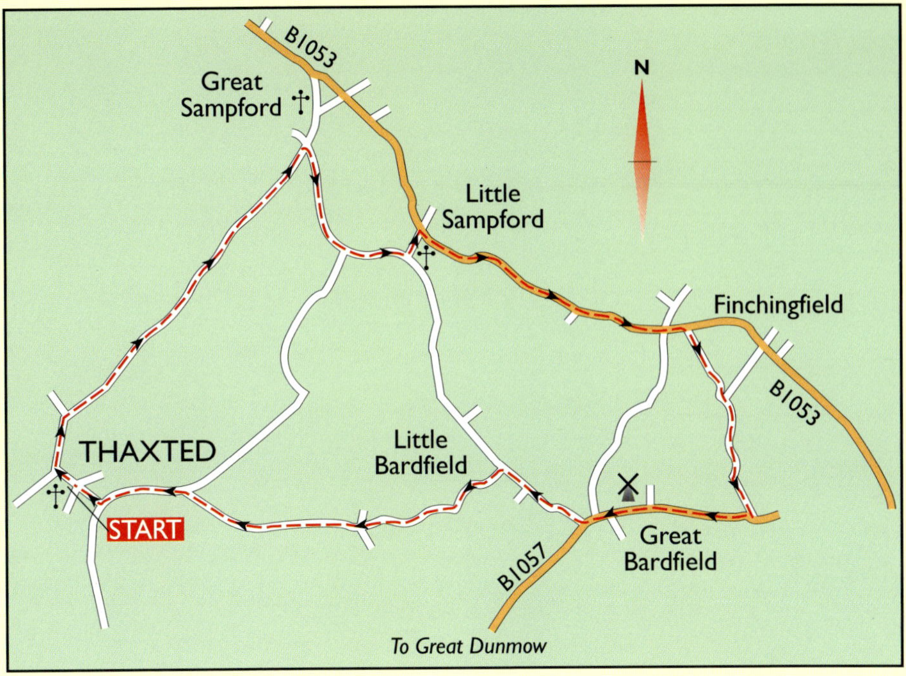

spread out in front of you. The Fox is on your left, the church is opposite and there is a green to relax on.

Continue down and across the bridge, up past the church and the Red Lion. At the Three Tuns **turn R** into Vicarage Road. Carry on along this little lane bearing right. After a sharp corner **turn R** at the triangle, towards Waltham's Cross.

After 1½ miles **turn R** towards Great Bardfield. Continue along here, passing the windmill on the right, and down into the centre of Great Bardfield.

Turn R and uphill and then **L** onto the B1057 towards Great Dunmow

and then **turn R** off it almost immediately on the road signposted to Little Bardfield and Thaxted.

Continue for about a mile and at the fork **bear L** towards Little Bardfield and Thaxted. There is a pub on your left and a church on your right.

Continue straight along here for 4 miles until you are back in Thaxted. **Turn R** at the B184 and ride back to where you started.

● ●

THAXTED
This is an amazing place, so make time to wander around it. It was built on wealth created by wool merchants and cutlers, and its whitewashed Guildhall and houses

THAXTED
GT DUNMOW
GT BARDFIELD
BRAINTREE

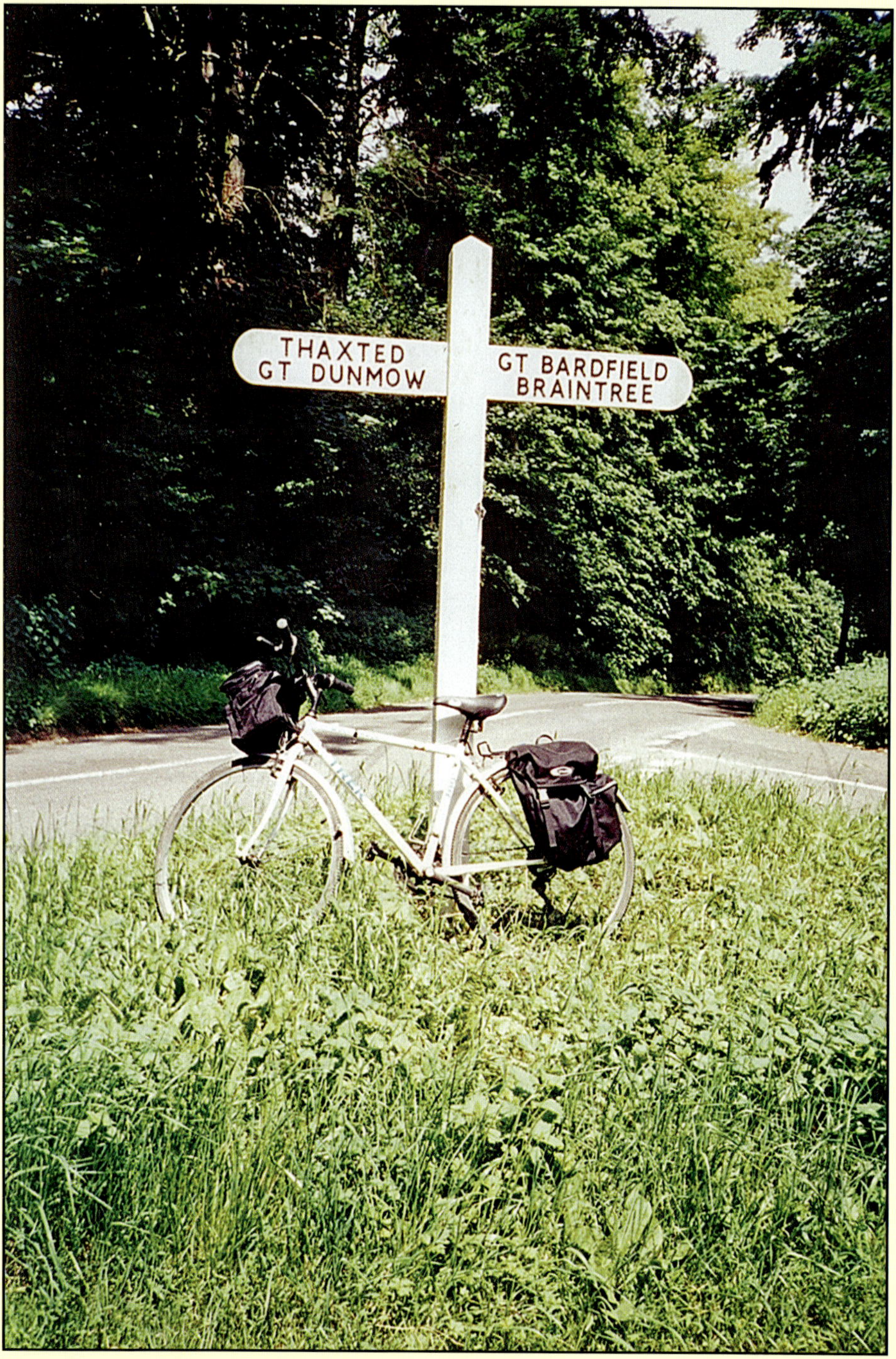

retain an air of solid prosperity. The light, high simple church needed to be big enough for the huge congregation that Thaxted once had.

One of Thaxted's famous inhabitants in the 1700s was Dick Turpin, the highwayman who has somehow come to be regarded as a daring rogue rather than a dangerous criminal, even though – or perhaps because – he was executed. More recently Thaxted has become a centre for morris dancing and in early June the whole place is full of dancers, musicians and spectators.

FINCHINGFIELD

If you think Finchingfield has everything a village should have, you are not alone. In 1951 the committee of the Festival of Britain declared it to be one of five perfect English villages, and since then it has always been popular. But it can't have been so perfect for the occupants of the workhouse (up the hill towards the church); they had meat twice a week and made do with bread, cheese, gruel and small beer. Nor was it good for William Kemp whose memorial is in the church and who lived at nearby Spains Hall. He accused his wife of being unfaithful, then realised he was mistaken and took a vow of silence for seven years. When seven years had passed he found that he was unable to speak.

GREAT BARDFIELD

This is another beautiful village with more attractive buildings and yet another interesting church. Don't rush through it.

Once it was the site of an important horse fair. Every year traders began to bring their horses from all over the country and from Belgium and Holland, arriving in time for June 22nd. Some of them took weeks over the journey, and it must have been an exciting and anxious occasion as they tried to negotiate a good price, and then drank in celebration or disappointment.

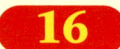

Littlebury, Elmdon and Chrishall

14 miles

This route takes you onto the top of Essex where you'll be impressed by the long vistas across miles of fields into Cambridgeshire and Hertfordshire. This is a ride of churches too, and of the thatched roofs of both mansions and dumpy little cottages. Apart from crossing bridges over the M11 at the beginning and end of the ride you won't see much traffic at all. This will give you the chance to enjoy the cloud formations above.

Hills on this route make it less suitable for children.

Map: OS Landranger 154 Cambridge and Newmarket, Saffron Walden.

Starting point: Littlebury church (GR 517395). Littlebury is about 18 miles south of Cambridge, and close to the M11. Parking is available for patrons at the Queen's Head pub, not far from the church. Please ask before leaving your car while you ride. As well as the Queen's Head in Littlebury, you'll find the Dial pub at Elmdon and also the Red Cow at your halfway point in Chrishall.

It has to be acknowledged that this route has hills. These are not steep, but some of them are long. The bonus of riding up each of them is, of course, the views. And it's only 14 miles.

Take the road leading away from the front of the church, signposted to Littlebury Green. You are riding towards and then over the M11. Then **bear R** at the first junction you reach, and then **R** again through Catmere End, towards Strethall (you can see Strethall church to your left). **Turn L** at the T-junction towards Elmdon.

Turn L at the crossroads and ride for 2 miles towards Elmdon and Chrishall. **Turn R** at Elmdon church towards Chrishall (the Dial pub is on your left) and ride on to a T-junction where you **turn L** and soon **R**, towards Heydon.

After ½ mile **turn L** towards Chrishall. Ride to the centre and look out for the Red Cow pub. Ride diagonally across the crossroads and continue until you meet the B1039. **Turn L** here towards Audley End station and then, after a mile at Wenden Lofts, **turn R** towards Duddenhoe End.

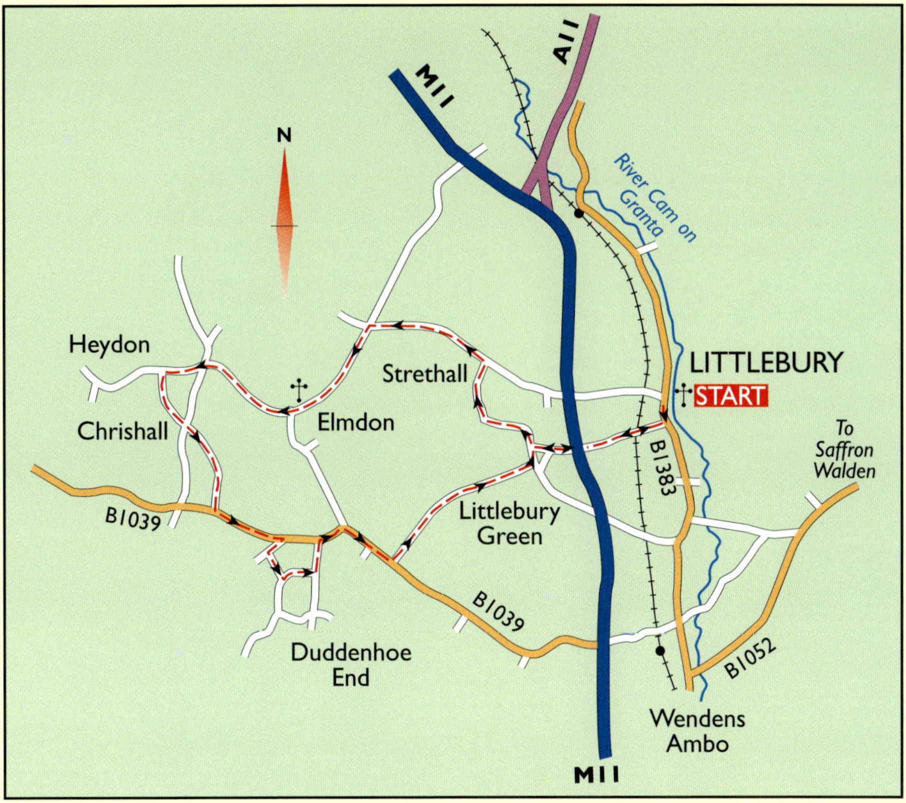

Ride up into the village and **turn L** at the first small junction, towards the Hamlet Church. Ride along, past the church and cemetery, then follow the lane you are on, round some bends, then **turn R** at the next junction and **R** again towards Saffron Walden.

Ride on until the turning to Littlebury Green. **Turn L** here and ride on and through the village towards Littlebury, crossing straight over a small crossroads and then over the M11 and back into Littlebury.

THE HAMLET CHURCH

Make sure you call at this beautiful little thatched church in Duddenhoe End. In 1610 the building was a barn, and it then became a house. But a thoughtful rector was concerned that his local parishioners had a long way to walk to church and decided to have it turned into a church. He collected funds from tradesmen and farmers, obtained wood from the nearby estate and involved local workmen in doing the work. When another nearby church closed down the Hamlet Church inherited its altar rail and classical marble font. It's intriguing to find a church where the altar is in a different place from usual

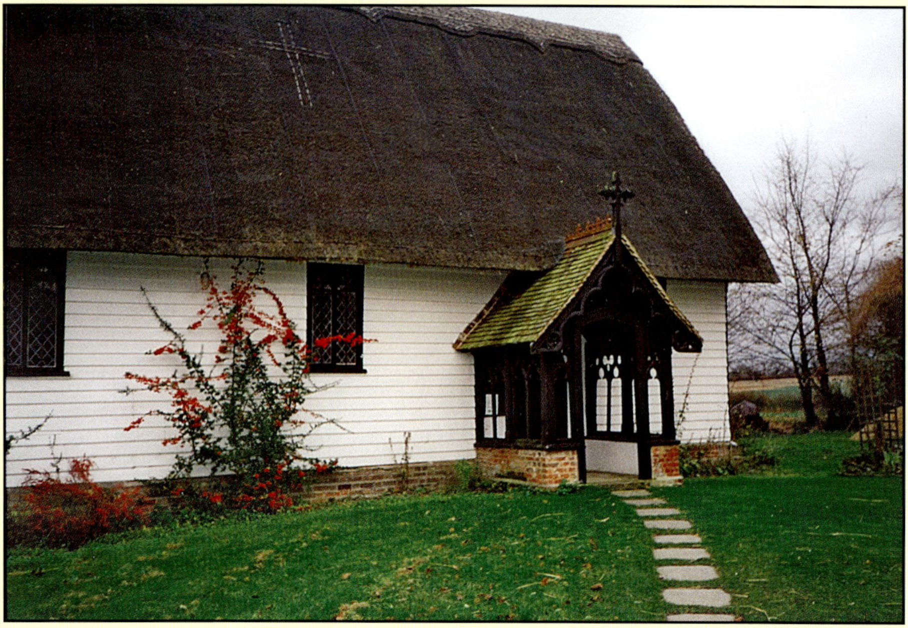

The Hamlet Church

and where the congregation face a different way.

THE M11

To cyclists (at least those on bikes, not those in cars) motorways are dangerous, noisy and to be kept away from, but on this ride you'll get very close to one of them. The idea for the M11 was first published in a report in 1968 from the County Surveyors Society which had been considering what a national road network should look like. The existing and expected economic development suggested that London and Cambridge should be linked and the contract for the first section was allocated in 1972. The whole project cost £61.3 million and the motorway was opened in 1980. The M11 has 123 bridges and tunnels (including culverts) in its total length of 53 miles, so there are another 122 waiting for you to discover them.

17

Hadstock, Saffron Walden and Linton

16 miles

This ride starts by the attractive green at Hadstock which is just south of Linton, a large village in South Cambridgeshire. The route takes you south on a B road past Audley End towards and through Saffron Walden, then up to the north via Ashdon and Bartlow as far as Linton, and then south again back to Hadstock.

If you are prepared to make a good day out of this it's worth spending time exploring Linton Zoo (but check opening times), Linton and Saffron Walden. Saffron Walden – named after the orange crocus which grew there and was used as a dye and in food and medicine – is full of interest. Lock up your bike and spend an hour on foot enjoying its little lanes and timbered buildings.

Map: OS Landranger 154 Cambridge and Newmarket, Saffron Walden.

Starting point: The car park at Hadstock Green (GR 558448). Hadstock is a couple of miles south of Linton which is on the A1307 between Cambridge and Haverhill.

There are pubs all along this route. Linton has three, but there are also plenty of cafés and pubs to pause at in Saffron Walden and, later on, at Bartlow.

There are quite a number of ups and downs, and some terrific views.

Leave the car park near Hadstock church and **turn L** by the King's Head onto the B1052. Now just keep steadily riding along for the next 5 or 6 miles through Little Walden, until you reach Saffron Walden. Although it's a B road it doesn't carry too much traffic.

Follow straight over all the mini roundabouts into town. **Turn L** at the big green on your left and onto Ashton Road. You'll pass the Axe pub. Continue along this road which takes you directly out of Saffron Walden past the Commercial Centre and along a more peaceful road between trees.

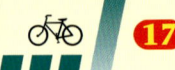
A1307

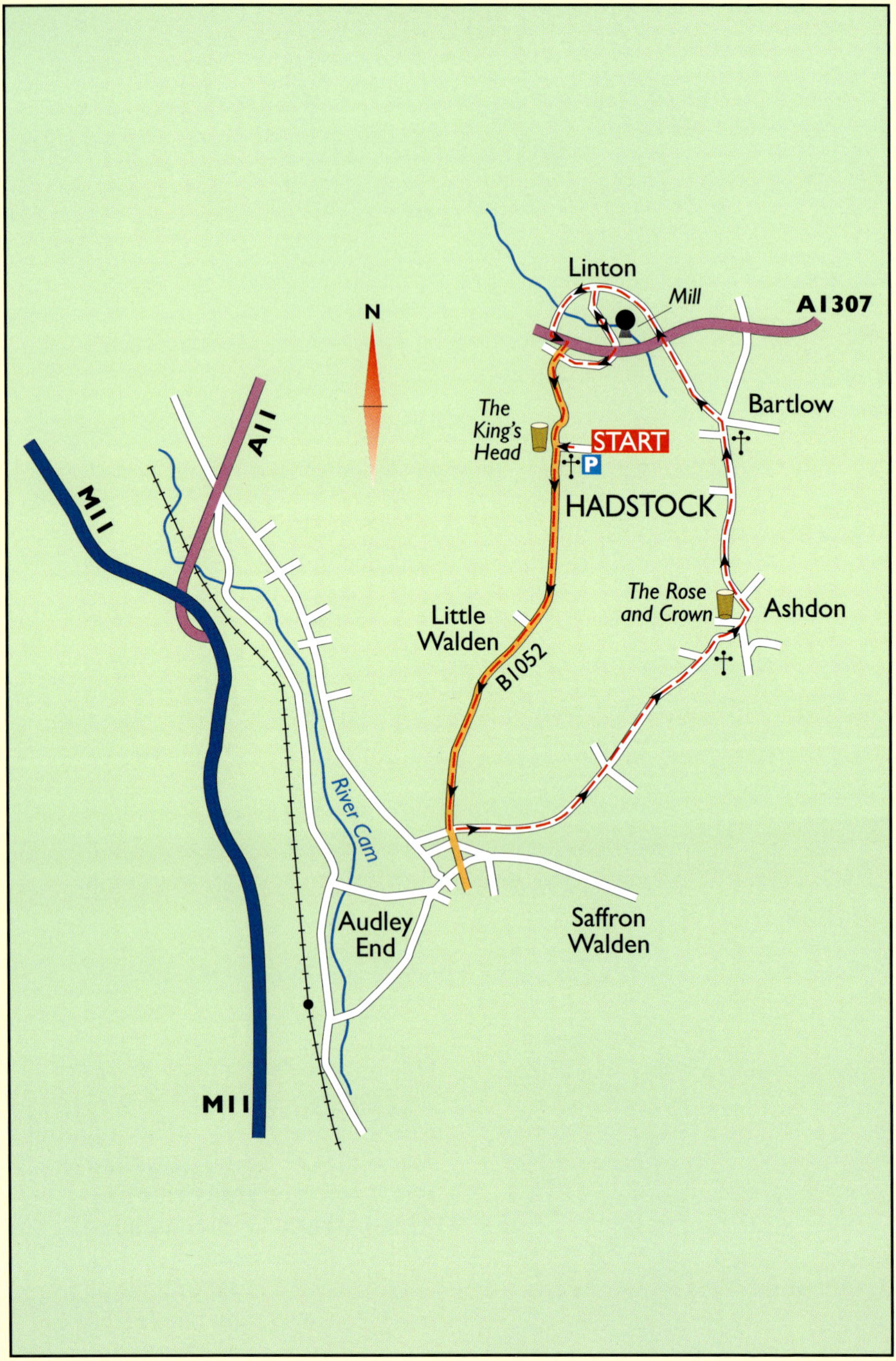

Linton

Mill

Bartlow

The King's Head

START

HADSTOCK

The Rose and Crown

Ashdon

Little Walden

B1052

N

A11

M11

River Cam

Audley End

Saffron Walden

M11

Just keep going now and after about 3 miles you come to the first part of Ashdon. The church is on your right and is well worth a look.

Ride on past the Rose and Crown and on into Bartlow and the Three Hills pub. Look out for the water tower over to your left, above Linton. **Turn L** at the crossroads and continue up the hill and along to a T-junction. **Turn R** onto the A1307 and then immediately **L** off it and into Linton.

Keep riding straight on into the high street which is narrow with interesting buildings. When you've passed the Waggon and Horses, keep your eyes open for Mill Lane on the left.

For a pretty little detour **turn L** down here to the mill buildings and the stream. Then go back up into Linton and **turn L**. You will soon come to the thatched Dog and Duck pub a little further on by the river.

Turn L carefully onto the A1307 and after a couple of hundred yards, **turn R** off it into a road called The Grip following signs to Linton Zoo. You'll see the zoo on your right. Ride straight along here on the B1052 towards Hadstock

● ●

HADSTOCK
Take time to look carefully at the door in St Botolph's church at Hadstock for it is thought to be nearly one thousand years old and the oldest door still in use in the United Kingdom. It seems that this church is built on the site of a monastery, but the village cannot always have been as peaceful as it is now, for the annual horse fair that used to be held on St Botolph's Day was annulled in 1872 by an Act of Parliament because it was so rowdy and debauched.

From the 1950s to the 1970s there was a flourishing troop of Boy Scouts here: the only mounted troop in the country.

SAFFRON WALDEN
This beautiful town is full of character and well worth exploring. It was a settlement in the Bronze and Iron Ages before being developed by the Anglo Saxons and because it has never been raided or destroyed by fire an unusual amount of historic buildings and streets remain in good condition. Wool was the source of its earliest wealth, then saffron, then malt and barley and, more recently, light industry and commerce. Although the church is the largest parish church in Essex, Quakers have played a vital part in Saffron Walden's history and the Friends' School in the town was founded over 300 years ago.

Amazingly, there are two mazes: one is a hedge maze in Bridge End Gardens, the other a turf maze by the common near the castle. If you're weary of cycling, a maze might be a good place to unwind – or wind up.

ASHDON
In 1865 Ashdon had a railway service and it lasted a hundred years. But plenty of travellers had already passed through the village on horseback or on foot. They included Oliver Cromwell and his supporters, one or some of whom painted pictures on the wall of the Rose and Crown pub. These are still there now.

Ashdon used to be a community based

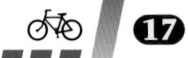

on agriculture and in the early 1900s some of the farmworkers complained about their poor wages and conditions of work. They went on strike and eight of them were briefly imprisoned in Cambridge because they refused to pay the fines imposed on them. This North Essex Strike was resolved with a compromise, but its value to the workers was diminished by the onset of the First World War.

Widdington, Manuden and Clavering

22 miles

This ride starts off in an ancient village with a famous medieval barn, takes you under the M11 and then off and away between spacious fields, past huge, solid houses and within sight of several particularly attractive little churches. Once the backbone of rural Essex, it's now desirable commuter country, but this ride takes you past reminders of those who lived here centuries ago. Even the placenames are intriguing: Ugley, Manuden, Wicken Bonhunt.

This ride is not a good one for children: it's the longest in the book, there are a few long hauls up and a half mile stretch of the busy B1383 needs to be covered twice.

Map: OS Landranger 167 Chelmsford, Harlow and Bishop's Stortford.

Starting point: The Fleur-de-Lys pub in Widdington (GR 538318). Widdington is about 8 miles north-east of Bishop's Stortford. Parking is available at the pub for patrons (please ask before leaving your car while you ride).

You start and finish at a pub and there are more en route: the Yew Tree Inn at Manuden, the Cricketers at Wicken Bonhunt, and the Cricketers Arms at Rickling Green.

You will not be able to ignore the hills on this route, but don't fret. Just get to the top in your own good time.

Turn L out of the pub car park and follow the road round to the right (opposite a sign saying Wood End) and into Hollow Road. Then enjoy a longish downward spin, but take care because this is a narrow lane. Go under the railway bridge and then **turn L** onto a slightly larger road that runs parallel with the M11 on your right.

Keep going along here for a good 2 miles and then **turn R** under the M11 and on past Ugley church which you can see on your left. When you meet the B1383 **turn R** by the Chequers and ride carefully along this busy road and **turn L** at the first opportunity.

Ride into Rickling Green and **turn sharp L** towards Manuden, on a

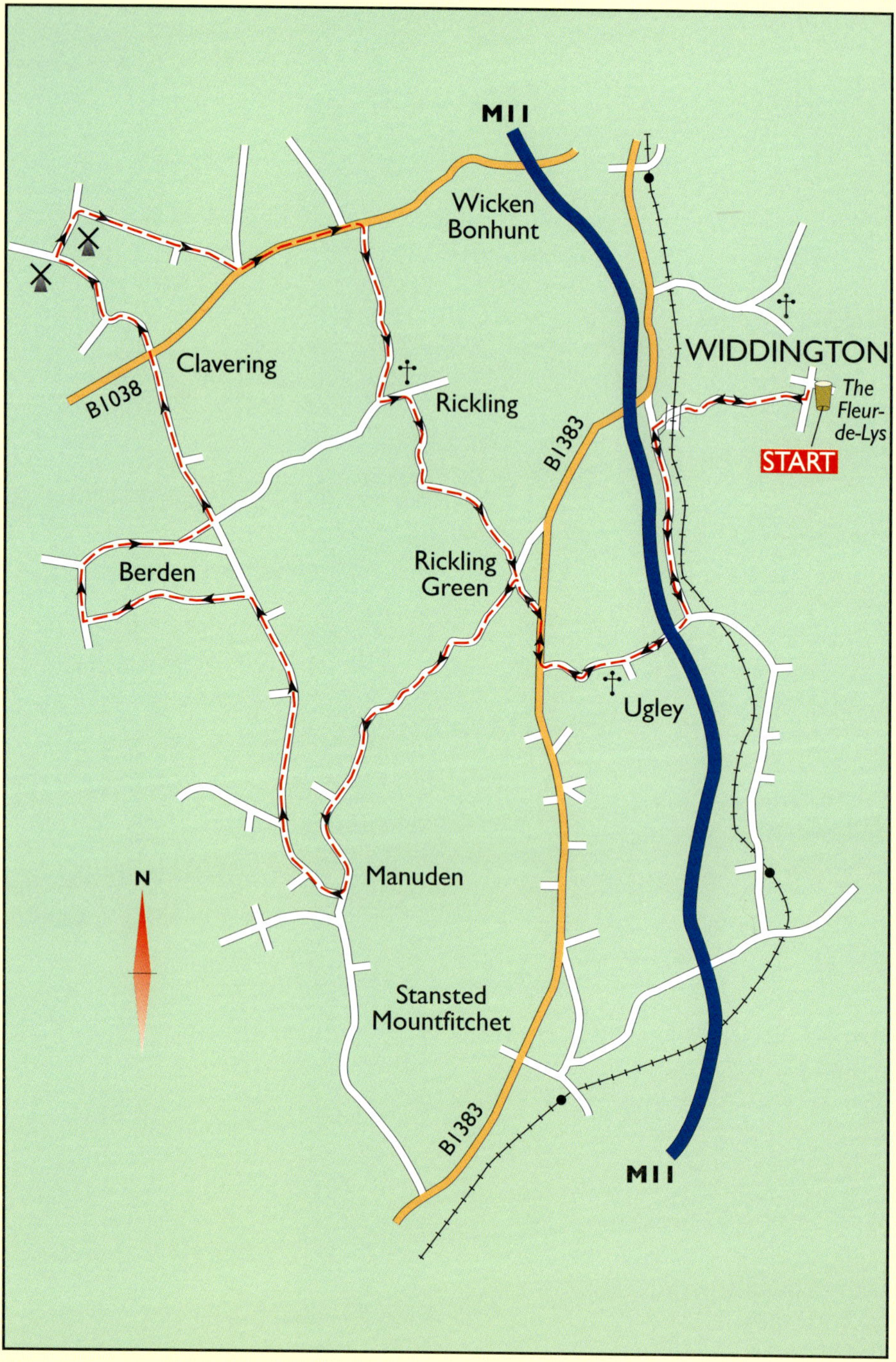

M11

Wicken
Bonhunt

WIDDINGTON

Clavering

B1038

Rickling

B1383

The
Fleur-
de-Lys

START

Berden

Rickling
Green

Ugley

N

Manuden

Stansted
Mountfitchet

B1383

M11

lane marked 'For Light Vehicles Only'. Continue along here for at least 3 miles until you descend into Manuden past the Hall. The church is on your left, the Yew Tree Inn on your right. **Bear R** and take the road to Clavering.

After 3 miles **turn L** towards Little London. Carry on and **turn R** at the T-junction and into Berden. You will pass Berden Hall and the church. **Turn R** at the next T-junction and then **bear L** at the fork. **Turn L** at the crossroads (and under the pylons) towards Clavering.

When you reach the T-junction at Clavering, you might want to visit the Fox and Hounds situated a little way along the B1038 to your right, but to continue you need to return to the crossroads at the point where you entered Clavering and cross straight over (from the Manuden side) and ride down to a ford.

Ride through or across this (bear right towards Langley) and then **turn L** and follow the road towards the two former windmills ahead. **Turn R** by the first and pass the second (on your right) as you make for Stickling Green. At the T-junction **turn R** and then **L** by the Cricketers onto the B1038 towards Wicken Bonhunt and Newport.

After a mile or so you are in Wicken Bonhunt. **Turn R** towards Rickling, and continue along, past Rickling church, and on for a couple of miles to Rickling Green. Facing the green

with its cricket square is the Cricketers Arms. Carry straight on towards Ugley and Bishop's Stortford. You are now retracing the route you were on at the beginning of the ride.

When you reach the B1383 **turn R** and then **L** by the Chequers. Ride back the way you came, going under the M11. Then **turn L** and ride along until you **turn R** under the railway bridge and then back up a steepish hill to Widdington. **Turn L** as you come into the village and the Fleur-de-Lys is on your right.

• •

WIDDINGTON

This village is famous because of the Priors Hall Barn which stands only a few hundred yards away from the pub where your ride begins. It's vast, and many of its timbers are original. Apparently, before the barn was built, William the Conqueror gave the Widdington estate to a French priory because its prior had given him his support. Consequently a French religious community came to the village to manage the estate but it ended up in the ownership of William of Wykeham, who introduced many improvements. One of these seems to have been having the barn built. Now Priors Hall Barn is managed by English Heritage, but check opening times with the Tourist Information Centre if you want to see inside.

BERDEN

Today Berden appears to be an attractive but ordinary village. It has a long history. In 1907 workmen dug up a human skeleton and items believed to be from a

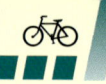

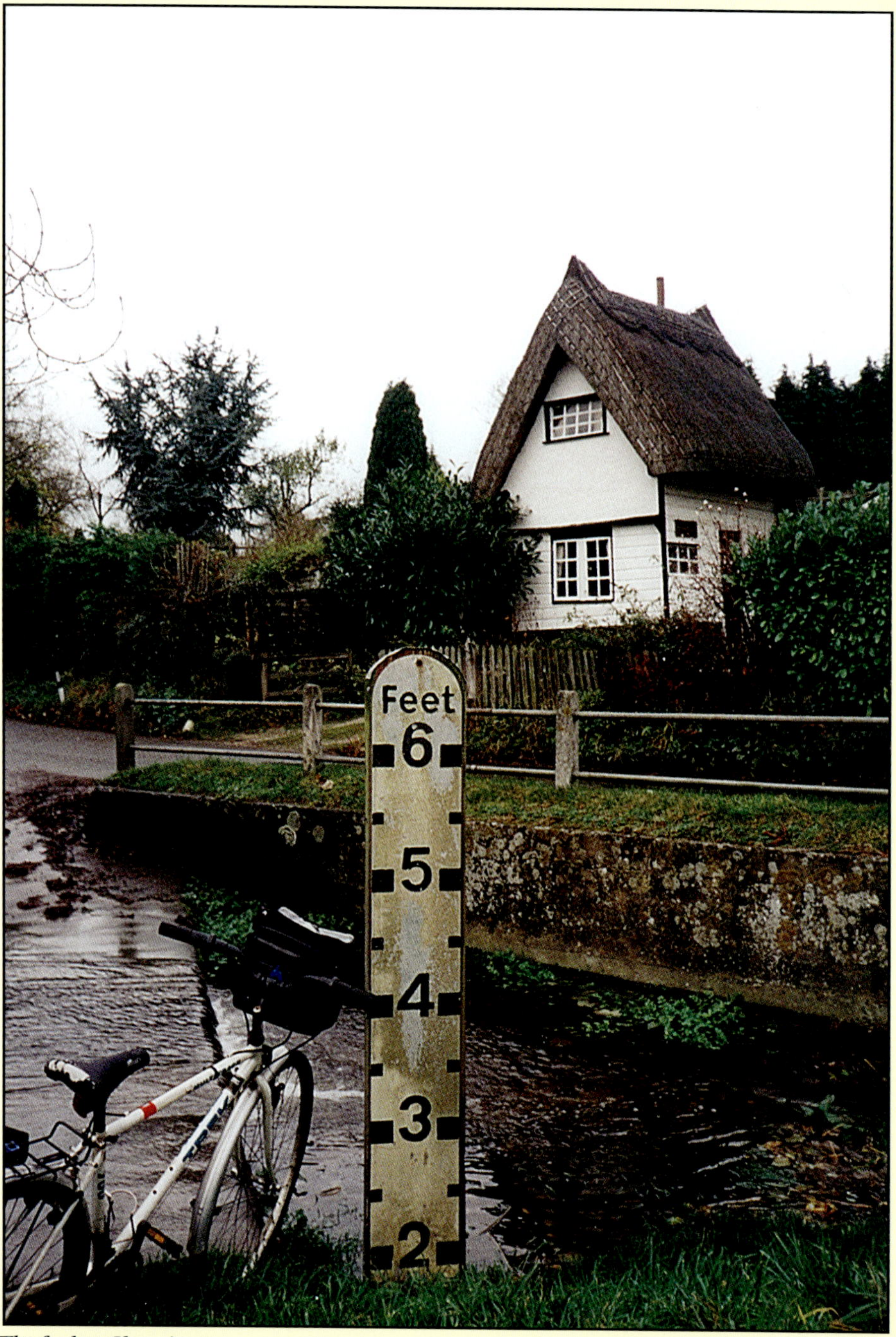

The ford at Clavering

Bronze Age burial mound. Roman remains have also been discovered (you can see Roman tiles in the fabric of the church wall), and an Augustinian priory was founded here 800 years ago. The Priory, a private house, was built on its site during the Tudor period, and Berden Hall, which you ride past, dates from 1580.

If you explore Berden a little you will find more recent reminders of commerce on the front of a building in the main street.

Ongar, Moreton and The Matchings

19 miles

Some people know this place better as Chipping Ongar. But whatever you call it, no one would ever know that this rural ride is only a short distance from Ongar underground station which is at the extreme north-eastern end of the Central Line: you can go straight from here to Oxford Circus without changing – an amazing thought. This route includes some delicious villages and wide miles of arable farmland.

Map: OS Landranger 167 Chelmsford, Harlow and Bishop's Stortford.

Starting point: Ongar Leisure Centre car park, just north of the town on the B184 through an entrance to The Gables (GR 552043). Ongar, or Chipping Ongar, is about 10 miles west of Chelmsford. Parking is free at the Leisure Centre.

There are various places to eat in Ongar but you may find it difficult to resist the attractive looking pubs you pass en route. There are two in Moreton, and you will see the John Barleycorn, and the Fox in Matching Tye and the Chequers in Matching Green.

This route has gentle ups and downs across rolling country.

Ride out of the car park and **turn L** onto the B184 and then **R** on the road signposted to Moreton. You ride away from Ongar along a road lined with houses.

Keep going along here for about 4 miles until you come into Moreton over the little bridge. **Turn L** at the T-junction and follow the road round to the left, passing the White Horse and the Nag's Head.

Ride on for about a mile and **bear R** up a small lane, towards High Laver. Pass Moreton Mill (Dalgety's) and then **turn L**, still towards High Laver.

Just after the church at High Laver, cross over the crossroads and ride on towards Magdalen Laver. Continue for 2 more miles.

Then **bear R** at the junction signposted to Harlow. Ride on past the John Barleycorn pub. Then **turn R** up New Way Lane and ride

on for 2 miles. **Turn L** at the T-junction and on for a few hundred yards. **Turn R** and then **R** again, following signs to Matching Tye, with its tiny green and the Fox pub.

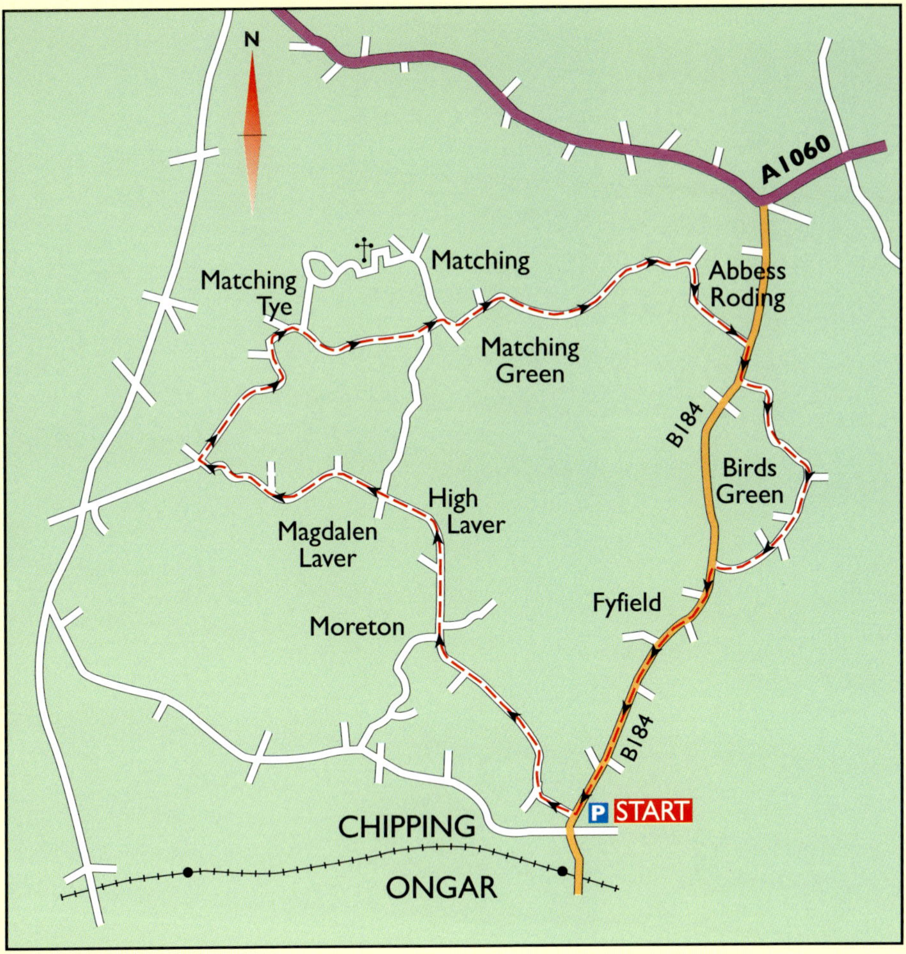

Continue through the village, following signs to Matching Green. When you reach the big green here, carry straight on (but note that a small road to your right takes you to the Chequers pub) to the T-junction on the far side. **Turn R** here and then **L** by the pond on a road signposted to Matching airfield.

Ride on along a road that crosses the former airfield and on for several miles towards Abbess Roding. You pass a driveway to Rookwood Hall on your right. Keep going, ignoring a turning to White Roding and riding on for another mile or so until you reach a turning

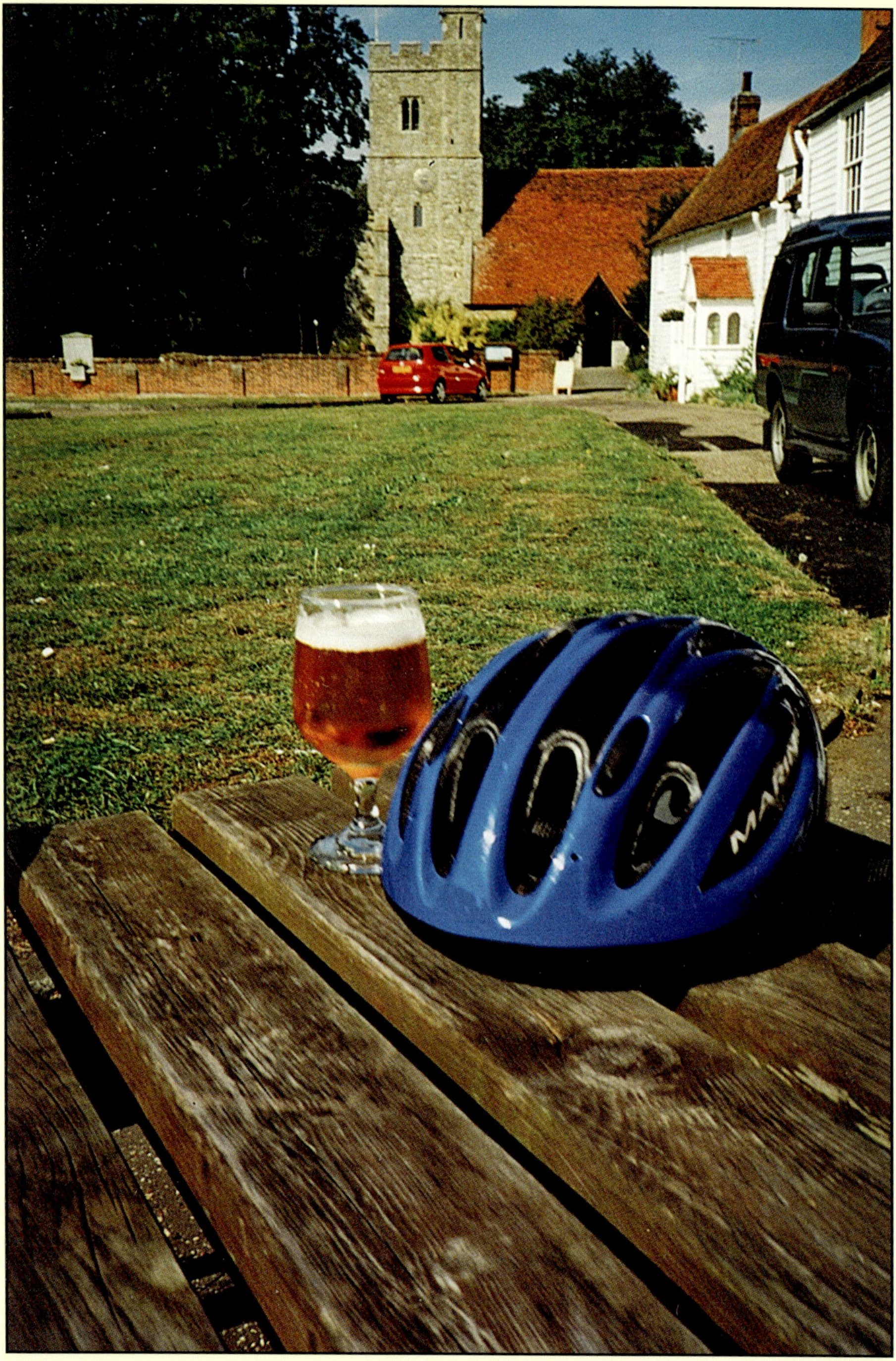

![The pub at Matching Tye]

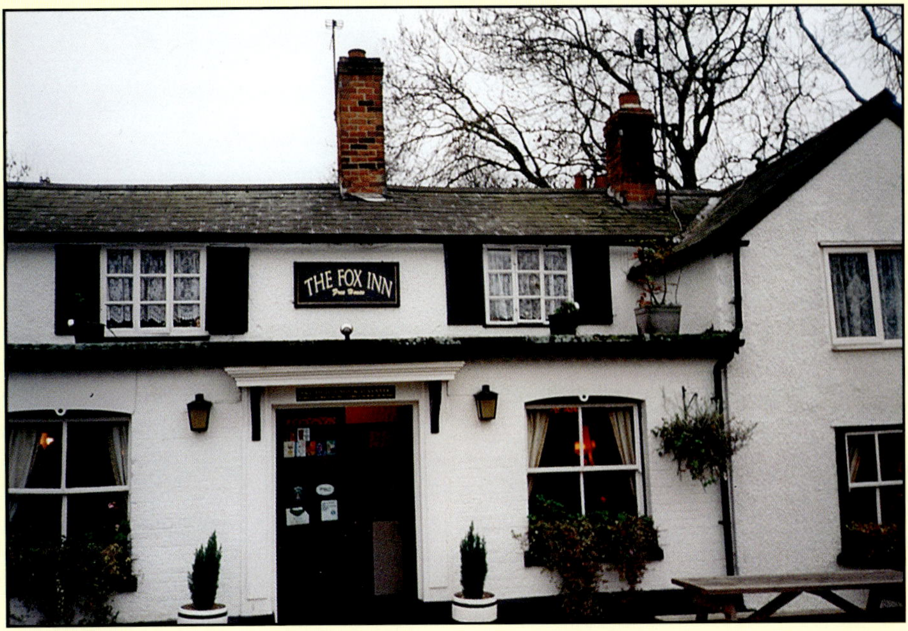

The pub at Matching Tye

for Abbess Roding. **Turn R** here.

You pass the church on your right and bear **L** here towards Fyfield. Continue to the B184. **Turn R** onto this road and ride for ½ mile. **Turn L** towards Beauchamp Roding and follow on for several miles and into and through Birds Green.

Ride for another 2 miles until you reach the B184 again. **Turn L** onto it and ride straight through Fyfield and down into Ongar. The Leisure Centre is about 3 miles from Fyfield.

• •

MATCHING TYE AND MATCHING GREEN

The Tye and the Green are just two parts of the original village of Matching whose

church stands a little further north than this route takes you. A building by the church is famous because a Mr Chimney built what looks like a row of terraced cottages but in fact the entire upper storey is one big room, a 'wedding-feast room'. Not many villages had anywhere big enough for plenty of wedding guests, so this Wedding Feast House is special.

Both Matching Tye and Green are very attractive although entirely different: one is a close and cosy intimate place, the other an expansive green with a pond to fish in. In the Second World War, Matching airfield was built for the US Airforce, and its control tower is still standing.

ABBESS RODING

Abbess Roding has two claims to fame. One is the tradition known as 'Watch and Ward', which started when Saxon kings

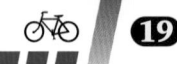

wanted to prove that they were in control. A special stick, known as the Wardstaff, was cut from Abbess Roding wood and presented to the Lord of Rookwood Manor. Then it was taken to Long Barns (a nearby barn) and all the local landowners had to bring the men they would provide to the king in a time of war. The Wardstaff was marked before being passed on to another community for the same process.

The other unique feature of Abbess Roding was its Anchor House, which is still there. It used to be an inn that was set up by the chapel trustees to serve refreshments for people between services.

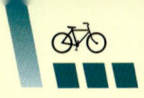

20

Epping Forest

11 miles

This ride is the closest one to London, but you wouldn't know it. It leads through the beautiful leafy forest, then north under the M25 and into parkland, then within sight of the ruined but still amazing Copped Hall. This is the shortest ride in the book so you should enrich it by setting time aside to take a couple of walks. You will see plenty of horses here, but they won't be bearing huntsmen chasing deer, boar or foxes as they would have done in the past, when Epping Forest was very much bigger and wilder.

All in all this ride is not a good one for children because it includes hills and some short stretches of busy roads.

Maps: OS Landranger 167 Chelmsford, Harlow and Bishop's Stortford and 177 East London, Billericay and Gravesend.

Starting point: Epping Forest Information Centre (GR 413981). Epping Forest is just south of Epping and just west of Loughton. Epping is 6 miles south of Harlow. There is a car park at the Information Centre.

The forest itself has more than its fair share of good pubs – such as the Owl and the King's Oak – as well as popular tea huts, and on the part of the route that takes you away from the forest you will find a few more.

There are hills, but there are more good swoops down than climbs up.

Ride out of the drive from the Information Centre and **turn R** and then **L** by the High Beach tea hut. The King's Oak pub is on your left.

Turn L opposite Arabin House and ride past High Beach church. Then **turn R** at the T-junction and then **L** at the crossroads towards Lippitts Hill. At Wallsgrove House **bear L** and follow the road down past big

houses and round a sharp bend and past a Montessori School.

Then ride uphill and between the Metropolitan Police Firearms Training Centre (on your left) and the Owl pub (on your right). **Keep L** at the next junction, signposted towards Sewardstone.

When you reach the A112 by the Plough, **turn R** carefully and ride on

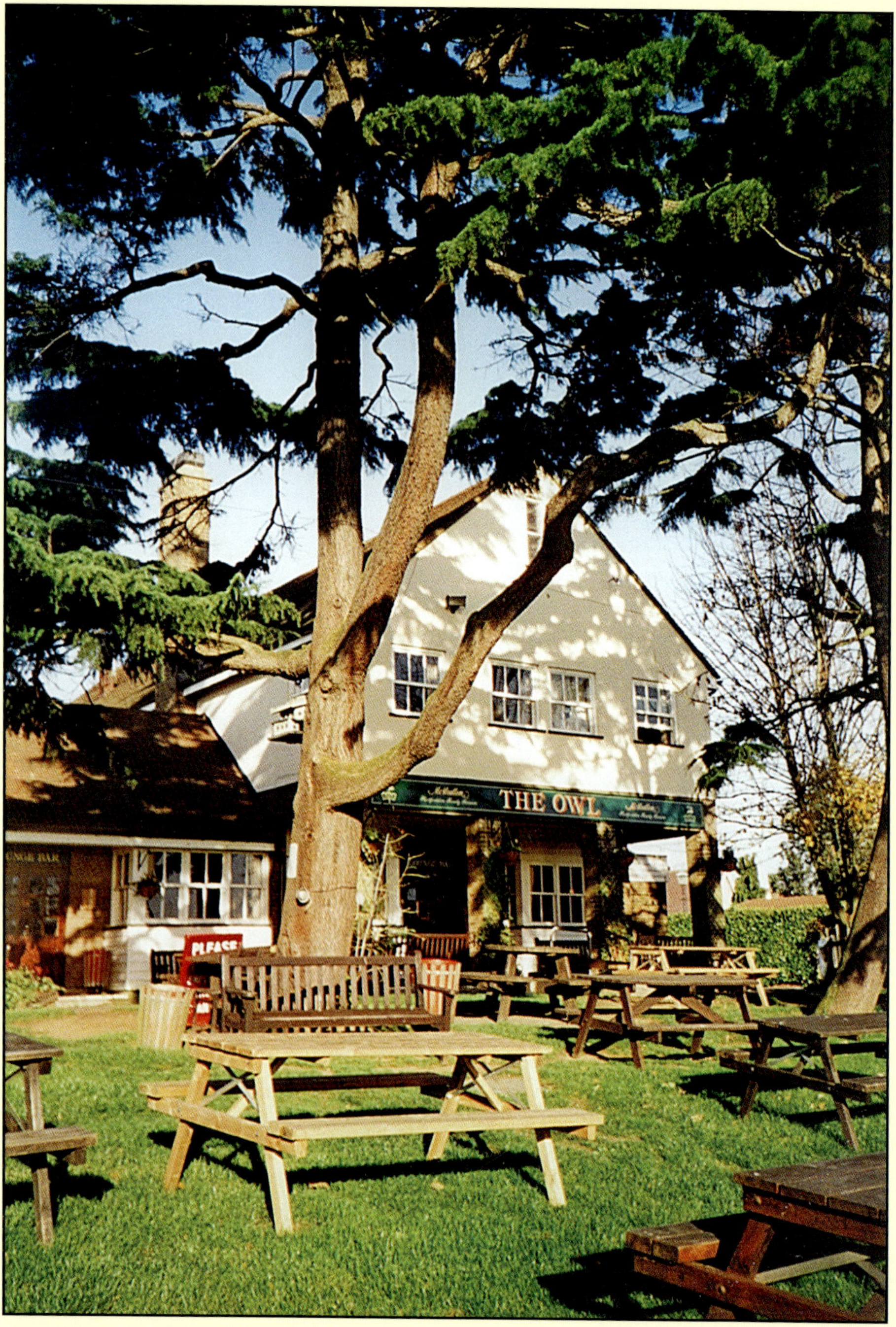

The Owl pub in Epping Forest

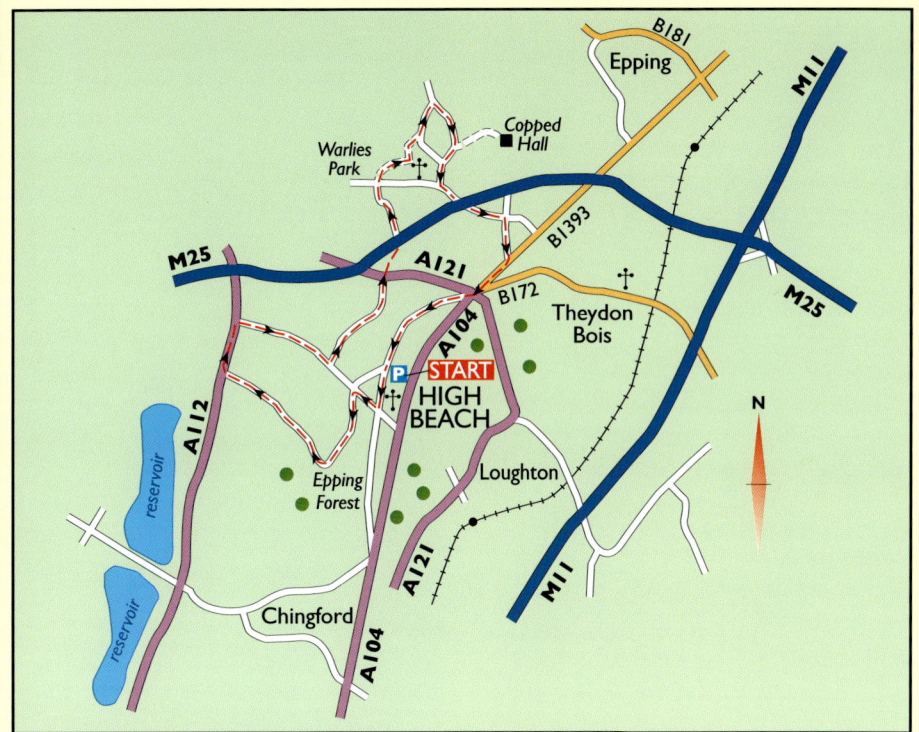

for about 1 mile and **turn R** into Avey Lane. **Turn L** at a little green, Pyenest Green, and **keep L** again and on past the entrance to High Beach House on your left.

Bear L at the T-junction (this does not look like a junction on the OS map). When you reach the A121 cross directly over it into Woodgreen Road. You'll see the Volunteer to your left and the Woodbine to your right. Ride under the M25 and on until you reach a T-junction.

Turn R here, towards Epping and Harlow, but after a couple of hundred yards **turn L** into Warlies

Park drive. Ride straight through the park and **bear L** onto a track by the entrance to Warlies House. Though this is a private road, it is also a public bridleway which cyclists may use. Continue until you come out on a lane by a farmyard, keeping a look out for an obelisk on a hill to your right.

Turn L here, and ride to a T-junction where you **turn R** and uphill. Then descend but look out for the lane on your left, leading to Copped Hall. **Turn L** here and ride up to the gate to the Hall, lock your bike and walk on towards the Hall. You'll get a look at it but unfortunately won't be allowed to enter.

Once on your bike again ride back to the road you were on and **turn L**, so you continue in the same direction you were going in before. **Turn L** when you reach the T-junction, and then **L** again onto another minor but busier road.

Ride down past the Good Intent pub and under the M25 again and then up a steep hill. When you reach an imposing gate and gatehouses (the main entrance to Copped Hall) on your left, **turn R**. You may need to push your bike round a tree trunk laid across the path, but there is a tarmac road here.

Turn R carefully when you meet the B1393. Ride along here for about ½ mile to the roundabout. You need the A121 (the fourth exit) and rather than going round this busy roundabout it may be safest to reach it by crossing over to the petrol station and getting to it that way.

Once on the A121 **turn L** almost immediately into a small road that leads into the forest again. **Turn L** at the junction and continue back to the Information Centre which is on your left.

• •

EPPING FOREST

The Corporation of London has owned Epping Forest since 1878, but before then there was a multitude of activity here that included Iron Age encampments, Boudicca in battle, stag hunting and holdups of coaches by the highwayman Dick Turpin. More recent visitors have been Queen Victoria, speedway racers, ramblers and school parties – not to mention the wildlife such as deer, squirrels, newts, dragonflies and jackdaws. The smooth barked beeches are lovely in each season, and there are also many oaks, hornbeams and silver birches.

You are allowed to ride on the paths unless there is a notice that says you can't, but Epping Forest is wonderful walking territory. Make sure that you have at least one quiet stroll in a glade or to a pond before enjoying a drink at one of the pubs or teahouses.

COPPED HALL

Soon after you have ridden through Warlies Park (once a Dr Barnardo's Home) you will see glimpses of the chimneys and roofs of Copped Hall to your left. There were people living in the first Copped Hall in 1150 and Henry VIII visited it, but around the middle of the 16th century it fell into a poor condition. It was rebuilt and Queen Elizabeth I stayed in it, but despite a succession of noble owners it was suffering from neglect again within 200 years so a decision was made to build a completely new hall and to demolish the old one. Around 1900, substantial improvements were made to this second hall, but in 1917 a fire destroyed virtually the entire building. The gardens and seemingly irreparable ruins are now owned by a Trust.

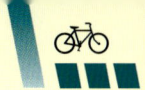

TOURIST INFORMATION CENTRES

Tourist Information Centres are full of useful, up-to-date information for visitors. All of them will provide details of their area and of other areas: opening dates and times of attractions, early closing days of towns, accommodation (TIC staff will make bookings too) and places to hire bikes from. Not all of them are open all year round but if one is closed another should be able to help you.

CAMBRIDGESHIRE
Cambridge	01223 322640
Ely	01353 662062
Huntingdon	01480 388588
Wisbech	01945 583263

ESSEX
Braintree	01376 550066
Chelmsford	01245 283400
Clacton-on-Sea	01255 423400
Colchester	01206 282290
Harwich	01255 506139
Maldon	01621 856503
Saffron Walden	01799 510444

HERTFORDSHIRE
Birchanger	01279 508656
Hemel Hempstead	01442 234222
Hertford	01992 584322
St Albans	01727 864511
South Mimms	01707 643233

NORFOLK
Diss	01379 650523
*Fakenham	01328 851981
*Great Yarmouth	
	01493 842195/846345
*Hoveton	01603 782281
Hunstanton	01485 523610
Kings Lynn	01553 763044
*Mundsley	01263 721070
Norwich	01603 666071
*Sheringham	01263 824329
*Walsingham	01328 820510
*Wells-next-the-Sea	01328 710885

SUFFOLK
*Aldeburgh	01728 453637
*Beccles	01502 713196
Bury St Edmunds	01284 764667
Felixstowe	01394 276770
Hadleigh	01473 823778
Ipswich	01473 258070
*Lavenham	01787 248207
Lowestoft	01502 533600
Newmarket	01638 667200
*Southwold	01502 724729/523000
Stowmarket	01449 676800
*Sudbury	01787 881320
Woodbridge	01394 382240

*not open all year round